THE ARCHAEOLOGY OF MEDICINE IN THE GRECO-ROMAN WORLD

This book teaches students and scholars of Greco-Roman medical history how to use and critically assess archaeological materials. Ancient medicine is a subject dominated by textual sources, yet there is a wealth of archaeological remains that can be used to broaden our understanding of medicine in the past. In order to use the information properly, this book explains how to ask questions of an archaeological nature, how to access different types of archaeological materials, and how to overcome problems the researcher might face. It also acts as an introduction to the archaeology of medicine for archaeologists interested in this aspect of their subject. Although the focus is on the Greco-Roman period, the methods and theories explained within the text can be applied to other periods in history. The areas covered include text as material culture, images, artefacts, spaces of medicine, and science and archaeology.

Patricia A. Baker is Head of Classical and Archaeological Studies at the University of Kent. She was made a Fellow of the Society of Antiquaries in 2006. She is an active field archaeologist and has participated in excavations in the United States, United Kingdom, and Italy. She is currently working on a project in Monte San Martino ai Campo, Trentino, Italy, a multi-period site dating from the Iron Age to the Middle Ages. She is author of *Medical Care for the Roman Army on the Rhine, Danube and British Frontiers in the First, Second and Early Third Centuries AD* and co-editor of *Medicine and Space: Body, Buildings and Borders in the Classical and Medieval Traditions; Practitioners, Practices and Patients: New Approaches to Medical Archaeology and Anthropology;* and *TRAC 98: The Theoretical Roman Archaeology Conference Proceedings 1998.*

For my parents

THE ARCHAEOLOGY OF MEDICINE IN THE GRECO-ROMAN WORLD

Patricia A. Baker

University of Kent

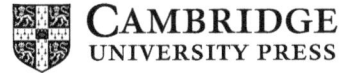

CAMBRIDGE
UNIVERSITY PRESS

CAMBRIDGE
UNIVERSITY PRESS

University Printing House, Cambridge CB2 8BS, United Kingdom

One Liberty Plaza, 20th Floor, New York, NY 10006, USA

477 Williamstown Road, Port Melbourne, VIC 3207, Australia

314-321, 3rd Floor, Plot 3, Splendor Forum, Jasola District Centre, New Delhi - 110025, India

79 Anson Road, #06-04/06, Singapore 079906

Cambridge University Press is part of the University of Cambridge.

It furthers the University's mission by disseminating knowledge in the pursuit of education, learning and research at the highest international levels of excellence.

www.cambridge.org
Information on this title: www.cambridge.org/9780521194327

First published 2013

A catalogue record for this publication is available from the British Library

Library of Congress Cataloging in Publication data
Baker, Patricia Anne.
The archaeology of medicine in the Greco-Roman world / Patricia A. Baker, University of Kent.
    pages   cm
Includes bibliographical references and index.
ISBN 978-0-521-19432-7 (hardback)
1. Medicine, Greek and Roman – History.   2. Medical archaeology.
3. Medicine, Ancient.   I. Title.
R138.B35   2013
610.938–dc23   2012050920

ISBN 978-0-521-19432-7 Hardback

....

CONTENTS

ILLUSTRATIONS

TABLES

PREFACE AND ACKNOWLEDGEMENTS

The study of medical history in the Greco-Roman world has led to some fascinating insights into how philosophers and doctors conceived bodily functions, illnesses, and medical treatments. Yet, examinations of the scholarly medical texts alone do not provide a rounded approach to ancient medicine; it leaves us wondering what the patient and general public thought about medicine and doctors at this time. We can also ask if there were different practices and treatments from those described in the literature. Fortunately, there is a growing interest in broadening the scope of scholarship on medical history to include conceptions of medicine beyond the philosophical tradition. However, accessing these views is difficult because many people in the ancient world were illiterate, and if they could write, they did not always leave personal accounts that record their views on health care or their medical practices. Nonetheless, there is one way to access a broader voice and that is to consider the surviving archaeological remains.

An ample amount of material associated with ancient medicine exists in the archaeological record, consisting of archaeological sites, structures, medical tools, votive offerings, bodies, and botanical remains to name a few. Still, there are very few scholars working on the artefacts associated with medicine, particularly from a critically interpretative position. Yet, as someone who works with many of these materials, I have consistently encountered two problems. First, there is an underlying perception that little can be determined from the material remains by those who work with medical texts (Baker 2002a). This is an unfortunate position because a critical analysis of materials can tell us a great deal about social perceptions that have gone unrecorded in writing. Second, I have also found that there are attempts by some scholars who have no training in archaeology to incorporate material culture in their work. This is promising on one level because it indicates an interest and awareness that artefacts are a viable source of evidence. However, some of the work demonstrates a poor understanding of critical methodological and theoretical approaches towards the remains.

Thus, two questions arise: why do such perceptions persist, and why are scholars unaware of the advances in the subject? I think a fundamental problem is that subjects are not made accessible to students and scholars in different disciplines. Therefore, this book is an attempt to do just that – to make archaeological methods and theories accessible to medical historians of the Greco-Roman period, from roughly the fifth century BC to the third century AD.

It was decided that a textbook that could be used along with general texts on medical history would be the best means of introducing archaeology to historians. This book will demonstrate the types of questions that can be addressed of material remains, and explains how the materials can be accessed and studied. It will also demonstrate that even texts – the main source of information used by historians – are a form of material culture. In so doing, it is hoped that students and scholars outside of the discipline of archaeology will be able to judge archaeological arguments critically and perhaps use artefacts in their own work, thereby enhancing our awareness of ancient medical practices and perceptions of the body and health in the past.

This book would not have been possible without the help and support of a number of people and institutions. To begin, some of the information provided about archaeological sites from Spain derives from a small project that was partially funded by a small grant from the British Academy. The staff at Cambridge University Press, in particular Luane Hutchinson and Isabella Vitti, was helpful and supportive, not to mention patient. There are a number of people I would like to thank for their support and encouragement: Professor Helen King; Professor Peregrine Horden; Lloyd Bosworth for his help with some of the drawings; Dr. Matt Edgeworth, Andy Hyam, and Gavin Speed, for their discussions about archaeology; my parents for their encouragement; Kate Tomas for seeing the possibility; and Dr. Sarah Francis for providing a good laugh.

I would also like to thank the two blind reviewers. Their insights and suggestions only made me more excited about the project and helped to enrich the content of the book. It goes without saying that any mistakes are my own.

Two people, however, deserve particular mention. The first is Dr. Neil Christie. It was through conversations with him that the idea for this book developed. He has been a supportive friend and mentor throughout my career and, and in terms of this project, he read drafts of the chapters, gave me the gentle and not so gentle nudge to keep writing, and encouraged me with the "odd" cup of tea. *Grazie tante!*

Last, but most definitely not least, I want to thank my husband, Dr. Todd Mei, a continental philosopher, who has found himself with trowel in hand in an excavation trench wondering how he got there and what is the meaning of it all. Fortunately, he saw the philosophical side to archaeology. He, too, read this book and provided unlimited support, encouragement, and help, for which I am most grateful. One of the great lessons I have learned from him is that when "life gives you lemons (or lack of understanding of archaeology), make lemonade", or in his case, a dry Martini with a twist of lemon!

CHAPTER 1

INTRODUCTION

It is incredibly important that the "small things forgotten" be remembered. For in the seemingly little things that accumulate to create a lifetime, the essence of our existence is captured. We must remember these bits and pieces; we must use them in new imaginative ways so that a different appreciation for what life is today, and was in the past, can be achieved. The written document has its proper and important place, but there is also a time when we should set aside our perusal of diaries, court records, inventories and listen to another voice.

Don't read what we have written; look at what we have done.

James Deetz 1977, *In Small Things Forgotten*, p. 161

1.1 INTRODUCTION

Not everything we do is documented in writing, particularly the routine activities of our daily lives, because records in both the written and oral traditions tend to be generated for extraordinary, unusual, and big events. The written record is, nonetheless, the basis upon which the subject of history, of all types, is investigated. Archaeological remains, meanwhile, can be studied and used to access unrecorded and mundane activities that have a significant impact on how people lived and understood their world. The aim of this book is to look beyond and behind texts and to explain how artefacts and structures associated with medical practices in the Greco-Roman world can be examined to determine past perceptions of health care, healers, and objects and spaces associated with treatments that might not be described in textual sources. It will be shown that archaeology is not simply a means of cataloguing artefacts and digging through layers of soil, but an insightful and critical scholarly discipline that can be used to ask vital and interesting questions about past lifestyles and social regulations that guided people's behaviours and, in this case, medical practices. The examples given in this study are period specific, but the methods and theories introduced through them can be used or adapted to study other eras in history. Scholars and students unfamiliar with archaeological data and their interpretation will gain an ability to make critical analyses of archaeological studies for themselves, draw upon material remains for their own research, and become familiar with the complex interpretations that can be derived from objects. At the same time, this book is a useful supplement to general introductory archaeological textbooks because they rarely contain discussions on medically related remains. Finally, some key recent developments in the field of medical history are presented in the text.

1.2 MEANINGS THAT LIE BENEATH THE MATERIAL REMAINS

Even when an unusual event is recorded, it can have a long-term impact that may eventually permeate people's everyday lives and prompt a form of behaviour that becomes a habitual and mundane activity where the original meaning behind the activity is seemingly forgotten. For example, Joseph Lister's experiments with carbolic acid as a sterilizing agent on wounds and surgical instruments have led to the common use of antiseptic, cleaning products in our own houses, bathrooms, and kitchens. With the exception of textual sources advertising hygienic household supplies, it would be rare to find a written account explaining the products someone uses to clean their home. If not in a third-world context, the lack of detailed texts exists because the activity of cleaning with certain items has become a common practice and something that is believed to be necessary to maintain a healthy – and civilized – lifestyle.

Social rules regarding actions and behaviours are largely realized and understood through habitual performance rather than through explicit statements. For instance, it is common for visitors to a foreign country to make a social faux pas when they are unfamiliar with the conventions of the culture. If a visitor thinks to ask someone native to the region why activities are performed in certain manners that differ from those with which he or she is familiar, specific explanations can rarely be given. In general, responses tend to be vague, such as "it is the polite thing to do" or "it is common sense", but trying to ascertain why an action is polite or a matter of common sense can be difficult. Medically related activities and feelings about the ill are also replete with culturally informed norms that are not verbally acknowledged, such as spacing one's self at specific distances away from the ill, keeping silent in a doctor's office, constructing hospitals in certain manners, discarding medical waste in specific ways, and fearing certain diseases and illnesses over others. Such reactions to the ill, along with spaces and objects associated with them, will generally vary from one society to another.

Yet, these are instances where "actions speak louder than words", since much of what we do, even in highly literate societies, is not described in writing. The question arises, how can we determine what life was like in the past if no verbal or written records exist that explain fundamental social customs and practices? It is here that the final statement of James Deetz's introduction to American historical archaeology, quoted at the start of this chapter, neatly summarizes the importance of using archaeological remains for the interpretation of past lifestyles.

It can be stressed that material culture, images, structures, bodies, and landscapes not only have a functional purpose, but, far more importantly, they convey rules and behaviours about the people who used and came into contact with them. Artefacts are, as Hodder and Hutson (2003: 33) argued, "meaningfully constituted". Conversely, they also play a role in shaping social conventions. Since anything manufactured, manipulated, or experienced by humans (landscapes, for example) both holds and shapes cultural perceptions and rules, these can be examined to access information about past routines and beliefs that are often not found in textual sources. However, retrieving meanings from remains is no simple task and requires a solid understanding of archaeological methods of interpretation. It is somewhat comparable to translating texts in a foreign language, also a difficult job, especially if the grammatical and contextual skills of translating are not mastered. When deciphering a sentence in a foreign language, one cannot simply rely on a dictionary to find *the* meaning of each term because the words, as any language specialist will know, take on different connotations that are dependent upon the context in which they are used. Grammatical structure, the society, and historical period provide a context by which meanings of words and phrases can be ascertained. For example, the simple statement "it's cool" can be used to indicate the weather or one's state of being. To establish which meaning applies, one bears in mind the grammatical structure, textual context, and the places and periods of time in which the phrase is used. Indeed, such words differ if an older person says them in comparison to a teenager. Artefacts also have similar rules of "translation".

Hodder (2007: 63–4) points out that while a comparison of finding past understandings of objects to a language translation is a seemingly appropriate one to make, he warns us that the idea of "translating" artefacts and structures is theoretically problematic, much in the same ways language translations can be. Translating artefactual remains, he argues, suggests that the explanations might be made to fit our understandings of the past, rather than the "past as it was". Our interpretations of artefacts sometimes do not account for the location of the object, the period when it was used, and, most significantly, different cultural perspectives and meanings that might be applied to the object. Thus, the archaeologist might apply his or her cultural views of an artefact in their interpretations. Hodder recommends that rather than seeing archaeologists as translators of artefacts, they should be seen as mediators between the past and present, who are aware of how their modern and cultural biases might influence their interpretations, and who are open to hearing the opinions of others. An example of an interpretation made with a strong cultural and temporal bias is found in some archaeological studies of Roman medical instruments that state that they were sterilized before use (e.g. Crow 1995: 50–1). Yet, this interpretation was based solely on the archaeologists' conceptions of how instruments were handled in the twentieth century rather than on the likely Roman conception of what constituted a useable medical tool. Roman doctors did not have the same perception of germs as that in the modern West, and there is no recorded evidence of them having purposely sterilized their medical instruments. Medical historians and anthropologists have shown that there are differences in the way that medical objects have been handled in other periods and places that do not conform to modern concepts of hygiene. For example, it may be more important to bless a surgical object rather than clean it in order for it to be considered effective. The Roman writer Lucian also gives us the impression that some doctors did not clean or care for their tools as we might expect, when he says that he would rather have a doctor with a rusty knife than a charlatan with a gold one (*Adversus Indoctum* 29). Thus, archaeologists are warned that they should take care not to apply their own common-sense perceptions onto past activities.

Despite these caveats, objects, like words, must be considered in their archaeological contexts to ascertain how people used and understood them. Hence, the methodology may be seen, in certain respects, like a critical translation. When writing about an artefact, archaeologists should make note of a number of its properties to determine one or more of its functions, to consider how people thought about the object, and to what extent it might tell us about social rules and behaviours for the period in question. For instance, a saw has many uses and could have functioned as a tool for carpentry or for bone surgery, particularly in cases of amputation. The tool's size, shape, decorative features, and the materials with which it was made should be recorded to help indicate which function it had. The archaeological provenance should also be studied to determine its likely context of use. Once one or more functions have been established, questions about the place of deposition and associated artefacts found with the saw can be addressed to determine other meanings connected to the object. Thus, a surgical saw found in an area used for the removal of waste could indicate that there were regulations about how medical objects may have been discarded. On the other hand, if it was discovered with votive body parts in a place known for ritual activity, this could indicate that it too might have served a votive role in a specific place and time. Hence, with the proper study of the material evidence, much invaluable information can be gained from them that would not be or cannot be found in textual sources; this enhances our understanding of past medical practices and perceptions.

1.3 RELEVANCE OF ARCHAEOLOGY TO MEDICAL HISTORY

Traditionally, medical history tends to be a text-based subject. Yet, to its advantage, it has much in the way of archaeological artefacts, such as instruments, anatomical drawings, bodies, structures for healing, votive offerings, charms, healing sanctuaries, and salubrious environments/landscapes that can be studied to establish past medical perceptions, healing practices, and conceptions of the ill. With such a range of materials available, it is surprising that there is actually little written on these topics from an archaeological perspective. I have noted elsewhere (Baker 2002a: 19–23) that one of the main explanations for this is the lack of interdisciplinary discussion between archaeologists and medical historians, which has led to misunderstandings about the ways both subjects are studied. On the one hand, archaeologists were not familiar with the medical texts, and, on the other, there is an ongoing perception that runs through literary-based subjects that little can be determined from the material culture. Archaeology is viewed as simply a function of cataloguing and describing remains, and to some extent, the interpretations are seen as conjecture (e.g. Salazar 2000: 230). Moreover, traditional studies involving archaeological remains of medical evidence tend to list the objects and compare them to medical texts (e.g. Bliquez 1981b, 1994; Bliquez and Oleson 1994; Jackson 1993, 1994c, 1995, 2002, 2005; Künzl 1983a: 15–29, 1996), sometimes without considering them in a wider archaeological context. Thus, an impression is given that little more can be done with the objects. On an even broader scale, although archaeology is very popular with the general public, misconceptions about the discipline persist because archaeology can be sensationalized in the popular media which focuses on big issues not everyday aspects of life. Details of the meticulous and complex task of making interpretations are rarely, if ever, presented.

There are numerous introductory tomes dedicated to explaining archaeology – its methods and theories – to students of the discipline. Yet, these
are not made relevant to specialists in other subjects. Since the basics are not
communicated, this exclusion will mean that the complex and multifaceted
archaeological arguments, interpretations, and scholarly debates will often
remain unknown beyond the area of study. For archaeology to be germane
to and recognized by other fields, such as medical history, then its complex
means of interpretation must be communicated with examples made relevant
to particular disciplines.

Another factor that contributes to the misunderstanding of archaeological methods and theories, duly noted by historical archaeologists (Deetz 1996
[1977]; Moreland 2007: 9–32), is how greater trust is placed in the written
word than in artefact analysis by those who are unfamiliar with archaeological
methodologies. This results in giving the written or spoken word superiority
over material remains. This is not simply a problem of text-based subjects, but
one even in archaeology itself. For the most part, archaeology is studied by
people who work in specific periods, as indicated by the division of the subject
into such areas as prehistory, classical, medieval, and historical (including industrial) archaeology. Although the term "prehistory" simply indicates a period
without evidence for written documents, a hierarchy was created when the
subject of archaeology was in its developmental stages in the eighteenth and
nineteenth centuries. During this period, societies with writing were deemed
to have more scholarly importance and relevance than those without a written
language (Schnapp 1996). In certain respects, this division is still maintained,
though there is, it is hoped, a growing awareness that societies without writing
in both the past and present have rich traditions of oral histories and complex
social rules. Groups without a written record should not be thought of as primi-
tive and, therefore, less worthy of investigation (Hodder 2007: 8). However,
certain long-established ideas can be slow in dissipating, as this hierarchical
disposition can still be found particularly amongst the traditionally trained classical archaeologists, who specialize in Greek and/or Roman archaeology.

It should also be remembered that, as with the interpretations of material
culture, the interpretative process particular to textual sources also carries
with it specific hindrances that need to be addressed for a critical scholarly
argument to be made. In the case of literature, an awareness of the possible
biases of the author, a fragmentary survival of the records, mistakes in tran-
scription, the social and temporal context of the author, and incomplete or
incorrect details provided in the texts, for example, need to be deliberated by
the historian. Hence, historiographical and textual methodologies have been
developed to deal with these issues.

Although there are different methodologies and problems dealing with both sets of evidence, archaeological remains and historical documents can be studied in tandem with one another. Sometimes the artefacts corroborate stories found in the written record, and, at other times, they can provide information about the past when no record exists, and they can even point to a different lifestyle or "fact" than that which was written (e.g. Christie 2011: 2–7; Deetz 1996 [1977]; Moreland 2007). Therefore, a well-informed, interdisciplinary approach towards explaining and understanding the past will involve the use of both documents and archaeological remains – to mutual benefit.

1.4 THE REASON FOR THIS BOOK

It could be argued that medical historians interested in archaeology simply should read some basic introductions to the subject. Those who truly wish to know about archaeology will most likely do so. However, many would probably find the introductions – to be quite honest – too dry and even irrelevant to their field of study. This is because there are few, if any, references made to medical history in general archaeological texts outside those that introduce paleopathology, which is the study of ancient diseases found on skeletal remains. During my first year as an undergraduate, I remember feeling disillusioned with introductory archaeology books, even believing that I might have made the wrong decision about what to study. However, once I began applying theoretical interpretations to the periods and subjects of my interest, the discipline came alive for me. Since archaeology is interdisciplinary, it related well to the other subjects I was studying: anthropology, classics, and history. It enabled me to ask insightful questions about life in the past that could not be answered through the texts alone.

My personal experience taught me that perhaps the best way to demonstrate the importance of archaeological remains to those unfamiliar with the subject is to make it directly relevant to specific areas of interest. Since then, my area of research has striven to bridge any divisions and to bring diverse data together. However, there is always much to teach fellow archaeologists: recognizing instruments as "medical" is rarely achieved; understanding the multifunctional uses of tools is poorly explored; discussing how both formal and informal medical practices were then, as now, an everyday feature of life and living; and how landscapes and structures also carry with them concepts related to health. All of these possibilities can be considered in much greater detail. To help address some of these concerns, for example, I have shown that the archaeological context of tools identified as medical objects have been recovered from areas associated with ritual offerings, indicating that the tools might have had a votive significance contributing to their multifunctional uses (Baker 2004b, 2011). I also found that the materials used in the manufacture of medical objects might have been chosen because the material itself was believed to have played a vital role in the healing process (Baker 2011). These studies demonstrated that medical objects can be thought about as having complex meanings that are not apparent in ancient literature. In a comparative study of the architectural design of medieval Islamic hospitals, I was able to demonstrate the interplay between structural remains and social concepts. Philosophical conceptions of healing might have informed the manner in which the buildings were constructed (Baker 2012), and conversely, the structures themselves might have informed philosophical ideas or understandings of medical treatments.

1.5 DESIGN OF THIS BOOK

Rather than writing chapters on particular methods and theories, similar to the arrangement of most introductory books on archaeology, I have decided to introduce these elements when discussing specific types of archaeological remains that are associated with medical practices. Therefore, this book is divided into chapters according to artefact classification: texts, images, small finds, structures, and archaeological science (e.g. human, animal, and environmental remains). Information will be provided in each chapter explaining the types of questions that can be addressed of the particular materials and where and how materials can be accessed, especially if the remains are unpublished. Along with this, relevant archaeological theories will be presented in a demonstrative manner through case studies, some from my own research. Each chapter will conclude with a list of further reading on the subjects discussed. Discussion questions and activities are also included at the end of each chapter to help the reader think more carefully about the issues presented and to create further discussion and debate about medicine and archaeology in the past.

The second chapter of this book will offer a general background to archaeological theories and field methods. The third chapter focuses on textual sources as archaeological remains. Papyrus fragments, inscriptions (public and burial), lead curse tablets, coins, and other inscribed objects are not simply items to be translated, they are forms of material culture. Some archaeologists (Deetz 1977: 24–5) argue that handwriting styles and language itself are archaeological because they are culturally manipulated and language, like material culture, changes over time. Textual materials, the foundation of historical research, are not only valuable for the information written in or on them. They also provide an archaeological context, or the fabric upon which they are written. The context where they are placed and stored, and even the artistic style of lettering, can tell us something about the way people were thinking at the times in which they were written. These latter concerns are rarely considered, but for medicine, as will be shown, they are vital for understanding why certain types of texts were inscribed on specific materials.

Images are the focus of the fourth chapter. In traditional Greco-Roman period archaeology, statues, relief sculptures, pottery paintings, mosaics, frescos, and images on coins and amulets have received the majority of attention in archaeological studies. The established approach tends to be art historical along with a focus on the narratives of the art object that are compared to textual sources. Yet, images cannot only be studied for their style and content, but inquiries can be made concerning how and where they were intended to be viewed and if they symbolize something beyond their narrative.

In Chapter 5, material culture is related to health care. Consideration is given to how material culture – also referred to as artefacts and small finds in this book – is defined, and how instruments and objects are identified. However, more insightful questions concerning the possibility of multivariant functions, deposition, and symbolism of medical instruments and votive offerings are also brought to the fore. The active manipulation of objects, mentioned above, will be considered in regards to healing practices.

Next, in Chapter 6, we move to structures, spaces, and landscapes that were intended for healing, such as sanctuaries, structures identified as hospitals, baths, and environments. The focus of this chapter is the identification of buildings, multifunctionality of spaces, landscape archaeology, and phenomenology. Included in this section will also be discussions on building amenities such as fountains, aqueducts, and latrines that contributed to people's heath in the past.

The final chapter focuses on archaeological science, including osteology and paleobotany. These areas of archaeology require specialist knowledge of anatomy and plant and mineral identification, normally supported by extensive scientific lab work. The skeletal remains can be used to make inferences about diet, as well as determine the diseases, hygienic conditions, and treatments people encountered. This aspect of archaeology also provides an ideal opportunity to discuss the problems of retrospective diagnosis. As regards medicinal remains, the ancient texts are rife with pharmaceutical recipes, but little information about botanical, mineral, and animal residues found in vessels surviving in the archaeological record are studied along with them. There are means of studying plant, animal, and mineral extracts in the archaeological record, so the latter half of this chapter will be used to explain how these are examined and the possibilities and problems of their interpretation. Since the ingredients used in medicines can also be used in food preparation, the problems of identifying when a food becomes a medicine, much in the way chicken soup today can take on both roles (depending on the context in which it is served), will be addressed.

1.6 LIMITS OF THE TEXT

All books have their limits, and I believe that it is best to state these from the outset so as not to raise the reader's expectations. This is an introductory text, and although I will be discussing a variety of important theoretical issues, these may not be covered with the kind of detail that would be found in more advanced theoretical and methodological books on archaeology. Archaeological interpretations are multivocal, and it is impossible for me to provide numerous interpretations for the information presented. However, I will demonstrate that there is a vast amount of untapped information at our disposal that ought to be used to determine more about medicine in the past than presented in the texts, and that these should be used with a sound understanding of archaeological methods and means of interpretation. In cases where studies have not been undertaken, I will sometimes give an idea of a question that might be asked of the material and offer a brief explanation of how the question can be addressed. Furthermore, as mentioned, there exist many archaeological remains of medical objects. Again, it is impossible to cover all of them in this text, so I have chosen a few key examples to explain archaeological methods and theories in relation to ancient medicine. Last but not least, the suggestions for further reading provide the reader with information about where they can access medically related archaeological materials. Some of these are not in English. Yet, given the book is written for both students and scholars, the resources are useful for higher-level study. Moreover, some of the foreign sources are bibliographic lists that undergraduates without a foreign language would not find difficult to consult.

1.7 CONCLUSION

In the words of Emily Vermeule (1996: 5), a classical archaeologist who was asked to give a talk to the American Philological Association, "[i]t is not easy to become a good archaeologist". This is true, since archaeology is not simply a means of digging up and cataloguing artefacts and finding sites, but is a much more sophisticated field of study that requires a high level of critical interpretation. Material remains are an invaluable source of information for learning about the past, and it is now up to the archaeologists to make their discipline fully relevant to other subjects. As will be seen, medical history is one that will benefit strongly from such academic interaction.

CONSIDERATION QUESTIONS

The exercise suggested here helps to determine how much you are aware of archaeology and the types of questions that can be addressed from an examination of the surviving remains in relation to medical history. It is not expected that the reader will know much about the subject; this is an exercise to commence consideration and discussion about one's initial knowledge of the subject. It is suggested that you keep a copy of your original thoughts to make a comparison of your knowledge of the subject after reading this book.

1. As a group (or on your own), think about how you define archaeology.
2. Discuss what you know about archaeological methodologies, what you know about making an interpretation from archaeological remains, and where you have learned this information.

FURTHER READING
Basic Archaeological Textbooks

Bahn, P., ed. 1992. *Collins Dictionary of Archaeology*. Glasgow: Harper Collins.
Gamble, C. 2008 (2nd ed.). *Archaeology: The Basics*. London: Routledge.
Greene, K., and T. Moore 2010 (5th ed.). *Archaeology: An Introduction*. London: Routledge.
Renfrew, C., and P. Bahn 2008 (5th ed.). *Archaeology: Theories, Methods and Practices*. London: Thames and Hudson.

Medical History Textbooks for the Ancient World

Some of these incorporate archaeological remains but do not explain how to interpret them.
Conrad, L., M. Neve, V. Nutton, R. Porter, and A. Wear, eds. 1995. *The Western Medical Tradition 880 BC to AD 1800*. Cambridge: Cambridge University Press.
Cruse, A. 2008 (2nd ed.). *Roman Medicine*. Stroud: Tempus.
Jackson, R. 1988. *Doctors and Diseases in the Roman Empire*. London: British Museum Publications.
King, H. 2001. *Greek and Roman Medicine*. Bristol: Bristol Classical Press.
Nutton, V. 2004. *Ancient Medicine*. London: Routledge.

CHAPTER 2

BACKGROUND TO ARCHAEOLOGICAL
THEORIES AND METHODS

2.1 DEFINING MEDICAL HISTORY AND ARCHAEOLOGY

In a book centred on the subject of medical history and archaeology, definitions of the terms must be provided. On a basic level, medical history is usually described as a sub-discipline of history concerned with medical practices
in the past. Being historical in nature, the majority of the materials studied are
documented in texts. It developed as a scholarly discipline in the nineteenth
century for students of medicine in Europe and America when the "great men"
of medicine and the long-term development of the field were the focus of
the curriculum. In the mid-twentieth century, the subject began to be taught
in history departments, reaching a wider audience of history students and
scholars. At this time, social aspects of medicine became the focus of scholarly debates. By broadening the approach to the subject, it became and is
still influenced by the theoretical trends and historical methods in the countries where it is studied. This allows the scholars of medical history to study
aspects of medicine and health with subjects covered in "mainstream history",
such as politics, war, gender, ethics, and religion, for example. Although the
approach to the subject always covers something medical, the boundaries of
the field are blurred. Medical history can now be defined as a subject widely
concerned with the body and health through time (Huisman and Warner
2004).

Like medical history, explanations of the discipline of archaeology vary
depending upon the academic traditions of the country in which the subject
is studied and the sub-discipline of the field, such as paleopathology, prehistory, or classical archaeology. Nonetheless, on a very basic level, most
definitions are quite similar. For example, Clive Gamble (2004: 15) states,
"[a]rchaeology is basically three things: objects, landscapes, and what we make
of them. It is quite simply the study of the past through material remains".

American archaeologists, notably James Deetz (1967: 3) and Brian Fagan, point to its association with anthropology because, through material culture, there is an attempt to recreate the history and functions of past societies. B. M. Fagan's (1988: 8) definition is more detailed, including understandings of ancient technologies, human behaviour, social organizations, and every aspect of human culture – something reiterated in Renfrew and Bahn (2008: 12) who say it is the "past-tense" of cultural anthropology. The definitions differ because there are numerous types of remains and periods of time in which archaeologists specialize and because each period will have particular methods suited to the needs of the subject. For example, an historical archaeologist will require familiarity with the material record of their period, the documentary record, and an understanding of historiography. Ultimately, however, a common element in all of these definitions is that archaeology is a discipline dedicated to understanding aspects of life in the past and uses material remains, structures, bodies, and landscapes as the primary sources of evidence.

2.2 A MODERN EXAMPLE OF MEANINGS DERIVED FROM MATERIALS: A VISIT TO MY DOCTOR'S OFFICE

The material world is all pervasive, and to demonstrate how it is important for conveying meanings and behaviours, I will provide a brief description of a visit to my doctor's surgery to illuminate the information that can be derived from material culture and structural layouts. Admittedly, the example presented is modern and British, but it illustrates how the arrangement of spaces and the material culture found in them are imbued with social meanings that are both determined by us in terms of how we use them, and, conversely, how they are determinant in shaping our behaviour. It also exemplifies some of the questions that will be addressed in the proceeding chapters. It should be made clear, however, that this description is not intended to be used as a direct comparison to Greco-Roman medical practices. The ancient doctors and patients would most likely have had different reactions to objects and spaces associated with disease and healing than we have today. Nonetheless, the material remains from the ancient world, like today, would have had cultural meanings associated with them.

The doctor's surgery I attend in Canterbury, England, is an NHS (National Health Service) facility. It was designed and built as a medical centre, unlike some centres which have been remodelled from old homes or offices. The approach to the entrance has both steps and a ramp to facilitate those with difficulties walking, as well as for the use of carts, carriages, and wheelchairs.

To facilitate movement further, the entrance doors are wide and open auto-
matically. Inside the building, the ground floor entrance is constructed in an
open-plan cruciform shape: a seating area is located to the immediate right and
left sides of the entrance; a reception desk is on the left side of the entrance,
just behind the seating area; the seating area for the nurses' station is placed at
the back of the cruciform, next to the reception desk; and a stairway, elevator,
and public lavatory are located across from the reception desk, just behind
the seating area to the right of the entrance. The patients – people of various
ages – are directed to sit in one of the waiting areas depending on the doctor
or nurse they are visiting. Those in the waiting areas are reading, staring at the
floor, or making cursory glances at others. If they are speaking, they tend to
do so in whispers. Infants and toddlers can be quite noisy, and their parents/
guardians compel them to be quiet and teach them the correct social behaviour by making shushing sounds. The lighting is somewhat subdued. Pasted
on the walls are brochures advising patients about screenings for certain diseases and illnesses, whilst old magazines are placed on tables for the patients
to peruse, and in the front area only, a few safe plastic and wooden toys are
scattered around for children; the toys have no small parts and can be easily
cleaned and make little noise. The patients are seated on non-descript plastic
or wooden chairs. Classical music, played at low levels, is sometimes heard in
the waiting area. There is usually a mild smell of disinfectant.

Once called into a doctor's or nurse's surgery, the patient is directed to
sit down, usually in a chair placed next to the doctor's or nurse's desk. On
the desk is a computer which has a database of patients' medical records.
A blood-pressure machine, blank prescription forms, pens, and a calendar
can also be found on the top. Other furnishings in the room tend to include
a sink, a countertop with yellow hygiene disposal bins or bags for medical
waste, and an examination table covered with paper, and sometimes a curtain
hangs around it. The cabinets below the countertop contain medical implements and supplies. The walls are usually decorated with the doctor's degree
hanging in a frame, informing the patient of his or her credentials. The music
heard in the waiting area is no longer audible in the surgery. Within the
room, a strict form of behaviour is observed between the doctor and patient,
played out through the observation of personal space, the layout of the room,
and the specific reasons when a doctor is permitted to touch a patient.

This basic description is replete with a diversity of objects and spatial
arrangements with which a patient comes into contact. No doubt the reader
can (and mentally will) add to this by considering their own experiences
when visiting their doctor. Depending on the situation, all of the senses are
stimulated to some degree; although taste was not mentioned, the flavour of

medicines can call to mind a visit to the doctor's surgery or feelings about health care. The objects and spatial arrangements enforce particular ways we are expected to think about medicine and behave in the spaces related to it. For example, the doctor's surgeries are closed because of a confidential doctor–patient relationship that is roughly based on the Hippocratic Oath. There is an expectation that the spaces are to be hygienic, which is met and indicated by the paper on the examination table, which will, we hope, be changed for new patients, the sink for washing hands, the yellow bags or bins for the disposal of instruments, and the scent of disinfectant.

The notices on the walls of the waiting area are written in a way to catch people's attention, usually in bright colours and/or with "scary" images that indicate conceptions about disease. Even though something might be curable, it is still brought to our attention as something frightful, alienating, and possibly painful. The doctor's degree informs us that there are standards set in modern Western society that doctors must obtain to qualify for the position. It also might give the patient a feeling of security that they are not being examined by a "quack". To put the patient at ease further, silence is observed; medical instruments are hidden and stored in hygienic conditions.

Much of what I have just described is often not recorded, yet we are fully able to "read" meanings from the situation and adjust our behaviour accordingly. Although archaeologists will rarely, if ever, have as much detailed information available to them as just described, they are interested in what the objects and spaces can tell us about people's reactions and behaviours in specific places and periods in time. Many of the objects I mentioned have a functional purpose, but there are often deeper meanings ascribed to them by the people who use and come into contact with them. For example, the examination table will be covered with paper to adhere to good hygiene practices. It may be shut off for privacy if there is a curtain around it, and is designed in such a way that the doctor is able to access particular parts of the body or to keep the patient comfortable during a procedure. Nonetheless, the sight of the table will also invoke particular feelings in the patient, such as a fear of pain or anxiety.

Medical tools, tweezers for example, may be used in numerous procedures including minor ones such as holding cotton balls, but in the doctor's surgery, it will be expected that they are kept in sterile conditions. Tweezers are fairly benign instruments, but others, such as needles and scalpels, may be hidden from the patient to alleviate possible anxieties about the forthcoming procedure. In another context, such as at home, tweezers are still used on the body, but will also have other functions. They are generally not sterilized nor are they kept in hygienic conditions in our homes. Thus, the context of the object dictates how it is cared for and thought about.

Such forms of behaviour are easier to detect if it is possible to observe people interacting in the environment, such as anthropologists do. However, without the possibility of first-hand observations, the main question is how do archaeologists retrieve such information from partial remains?

2.3 EVOLVING ARCHAEOLOGICAL THEORY

Before the detailed chapters can be presented, there are certain basics to archaeological interpretation that require explanation. Although archaeological theory is a subject of considerable debate (e.g. Binford 1972; Bintliff and Pearce 2011; Clark 1939; Clarke 1973; Hodder 1982a, 1982b, 1996, 2001, 2007; Shanks and Tilley 1987, 1992), some basics require explanation because the reader will encounter the topic if they wish to undertake further study on the subject. Archaeological interpretations of material remains are affected by the themes present in scholarship at particular periods in time. Not only does this shape how the remains are interpreted, but also how they are collected, recorded, and excavated.

Archaeology is a fairly young subject. However, collecting objects, writing histories, and making sense of the remains of the past is not in any way new, and evidence can be found for this practice in many societies past and present (Schnapp 1996). Thus, pinpointing an exact date for when archaeology became a discipline is difficult. One could argue that its methodology originated during the period of Enlightenment in the eighteenth century. At this time, European explorers were mapping new territories and returning home with unusual objects, animals, plants, and accounts of different cultures to document their trips and discoveries. To make sense of the objects they brought home, they classified them into the scientific systems that were developing at the time, which remains the basis for the way we categorize and undertake scientific research today. Hence, artefacts were organized in a classification system defined by fabric, design, and function, much like animal and plant taxonomies.

Artefacts, usually sculptures, fine painted pottery, and even structures, were also collected from places such as Greece and Rome, but the excavation techniques were far from standardized and many were equivalent to searching for treasure by digging holes in the earth. Thus, the context and associated artefacts remain unknown for the majority of items discovered and given to museums during this era.

In the nineteenth century, there were developments in excavation techniques that led to more systematic fieldwork than the acquisition of objects seen in previous centuries. However, the quality of excavation and recording were quite variable between sites. Ultimately, the archaeologists of the time were still in the early stages of learning to make sense of the objects and stratigraphy they encountered. As the century progressed, there were developments in understanding the stratigraphy found within excavation trenches and its relationship to dating objects. As the century came to a close, the publication of site reports became more common, some of which record the trenches excavated and the artefacts discovered in them.

In the twentieth century, numerous advances occurred in both field and interpretative methodologies. Theoretically, archaeology generally underwent three stages of questioning and development: cultural history, processual (also termed new or functional archaeology), and postprocessual archaeology. There is always overlap between these stages of development, and not every archaeologist will strictly adhere to one means of interpretation; some continue to work in terms of cultural history and processual archaeology in spite of more recent disciplinary changes. Most will probably use a combination of interpretative theories.

2.3.1 Cultural History

Beginning with cultural history, this interpretative method developed in the early twentieth century when archaeologists were still formulating excavation, dating, and classificatory techniques (see Trigger 2006: 211–313 for a thorough discussion). Questions addressed not only concerned the identification and date of the material but for which group of people it belonged. Most of the dating at this time was relative rather than absolute, meaning artefacts were dated according to their styles of decoration and their sequence in the archaeological record. Put simply objects found in a stratigraphic layer above a particular object were later in date, and those found in the layer below an object were earlier in date. The styles of an object found in a layer were used to form a dating sequence across other sites. Closer dates could be given to artefacts that were found with inscriptions and coins, but it was not until the development of carbon fourteen (^{14}C) dating by Willard Libby in the 1940s that more precise or what is referred to as absolute dating became possible for organic remains.

Besides dating sequences, questions about the culture of the people to which the objects belonged began to be addressed, especially in terms of how materials and ideas were adapted from one area to another. In terms of cultural history, social changes were explained by theories of invasion or migration. A certain design of medical tool found in Rome would, for example, could be interpreted not only as a Roman object but also as a symbol of

Roman culture. With this assumption followed an interpretative idea: when an object was found outside of Italy, then archaeologists tended to assume it was incorporated into the new region, say Gaul, through the invasion or migration of the Romans, particularly the Roman army (e.g. Nutton 1972). It is possible that this was the case in certain instances. However, such an interpretation has been shown to be extremely problematic because the Roman army consisted of soldiers from areas outside of Italy. So in hindsight, one can ask whether the objects were introduced by the soldiers, and if so, whether they were understood in the same way as those in Rome used and understood them (Baker 2004a).

2.3.2 Processual Archaeology

In the 1960s and 1970s, archaeologists began to expand their approaches to the subject. The changes that came about were influenced by the earlier work of Graham Clark (1939), who stated in *Archaeology and Society* that archaeology should be about *how* humans lived in the past. His work was influenced by environmental sciences and functionalist anthropology. The anthropological approach fuelled his interest in reconstructing social systems. The primary argument developed from this was that societies were chiefly concerned with ensuring their survival, which was basically a reaction to environmental changes. Like the ecosystem, Clark argued that societies were homostats, meaning they were self-correcting towards temporary fluctuations in the environment, such as drought, disease, or flood, and this, rather than invasion or migration, was the cause of social change.

In 1959, Joseph Caldwell wrote an article entitled "The New American Archaeology" in *Science* where he argued that there were a finite number of general historical processes in which all societies had to function. The goal of archaeology was, therefore, to understand these cultural processes. Hence, the term processual archaeology was born. Lewis Binford (1962), an American anthropologist and archaeologist developed this idea by arguing that archaeology was anthropology, and its main role was to explain the full range of differences and similarities in cultural processes. Like Graham Clark, culture to Binford was tied to environmental adaptations.

Another area of interest for Binford was the formation of the archaeological record. To determine how sites were created, he believed archaeologists could make comparisons to modern cultures through the observation of specific activities. He examined the activities that occurred at Inuit butchering sites and made note of the waste materials that were left behind. Then he compared these archaeological examples to non-modern butchering sites. This comparative device is known as Middle Range Theory because it helps us to determine how the archaeological record was created by likening the remains of artefacts with anthropological examples of similar activities. Although a useful means of creating discussion and helpful to archaeologists in identifying particular site patterns and activities, it can become problematic if an archaeologist assumes that the activities that occurred in the past were executed and understood in exactly the same manner to those being observed in the present, as pointed out with the modern example of my doctor's surgery.

In Britain during the late 1960s and early 1970s, David Clarke, an archaeology student of Graham Clark's, advocated that archaeology should be seen as a hard science. The use of analytic methods to determine social processes was encouraged. He argued that past social meanings and activities could be determined through a scientific hypothesis, which could be measured much like a lab-based experiment. His main objective was to develop a universal scientific framework in which material remains could be questioned (Clarke 1973). Nonetheless, the positivistic nature of this approach could only lead to generalized statements about societies in the past, and very little about individual groups of people could be determined from this methodology.

2.3.3 Postprocessual Archaeology

Towards the early 1980s into the 1990s, many archaeologists, particularly in Britain, became disillusioned with these generalizations and the attempt to use scientific methodology. The main objection was that, in certain respects, people and the actions of the people were being excluded from archaeological discussions, and when they were mentioned, it was almost as if they were being described like automatons or bees in a hive. Archaeologists, particularly Ian Hodder, realized through social anthropological studies that these methods were limiting. In his observations, he found that the use of material culture was far more complex than a simple by-product of broader social activities and changes. Objects, he and others found, carried with them numerous meanings and associations that could not only represent social activities but also had the power to transform them. He, and others, realized that material culture could be used to denote gender, age, and social identity, and could play a role in differentiating social relations. It thus became evident that there had not been a social study of symbolism and conceptual schemes that might underlie the use of remains. Postprocessual archaeology emerged from this. Yet, unlike the previous two "schools" of thought, postprocessual archaeology, or as Johnson (2000: 101) prefers to call it "interpretative archaeologies", does not adhere to a uniform theoretical stance. It consists rather of a variety of interpretative methods such as those concerned with gender and agency. Its uniting factor is the idea that positivistic science cannot be used to find an overarching truth about the past.

A range of theoretical approaches began to appear in archaeological interpretations following on from Hodder's initial observations. There was no longer a single view on how archaeology could be defined (Hodder 2007: 5). The emergence of this broader perspective towards archaeological interpretations has forced archaeologists to consider how their cultural understandings and practices can be imparted onto interpretations of the past. One of the reasons for this expansion is archaeologists have become more "self-aware" of how they are thinking and interpreting their materials. This new type of critical reflection can be called "hermeneutical", which means that archaeology is not only concerned with meanings given to the remains questioned, but also how and why these interpretations are made. Hermeneutics is essentially concerned with asking how we make our interpretations. The hermeneutical approach has helped to promote an awareness that multivariant cultural significances and underlying conceptions can be given to and obtained from objects. Moreover, the individual became a point of study and was seen as an active agent in society who informed the use and understanding of objects.

Hence, many sub-disciplines of archaeology now allow for multivocal perspectives. Nonetheless, some areas have remained more traditional in their approach, but this is not to say that the material from these periods cannot be examined in different manners, as will be demonstrated in the coming chapters.

2.4 INTRODUCTION TO FIELD METHODS

Having just provided some basic background information to the development of archaeological interpretative theory, it should be evident that actual field methods were not mentioned. From my division, it might appear that the two are mutually exclusive – this exclusivity might also be apparent in papers and books that focus on one particular element of archaeology. However, this impression is, in fact, incorrect. Both field methods and interpretations influence one another. Yet, to those new to the discipline, the simplest way to explain them is to write about each separately, and once the basics are mastered, it becomes easier to see the relationship between the two seemingly disparate activities.

It is expected that the majority of readers of this book may never put a trowel to soil, and because of this, field methods will rarely be discussed in the text. Yet, it is still vital that anyone who may wish to use published archaeological remains in their work or critically assess a work that contains discussions on remains be aware of how the information is retrieved and recorded. Field archaeology is not a thoughtless activity; archaeologists do not just decide to dig in a random place. They develop research strategies for undertaking excavations that are dictated by questions they might wish to address about a potential site. Since there are specific concerns, it means, to cite Roskams (2001: 30) "[d]ata are not gathered passively" but with an intention of asking specific questions. Therefore, some types of remains might be overlooked in the excavation and cataloguing process. The methods used to collect and record the data are, to a large extent, determined by the questions the archaeologist poses.

To present the reader with an idea of how archaeologists embark upon an excavation, a fictitious excavation is explained in Box One below. I have chosen to explain an archaeological excavation in this manner because everything I wish to discuss throughout the text is included here, where it might not be on a real site. Given in the example are some basic explanations about setting up a site, digging it, and bringing it to publication. However, being fictitious, the normal financial burden and problems of obtaining a permit for digging are assumed to have been sorted, though in reality these issues can cause great stress and difficulty. It is not always easy to acquire funding or obtain permission to work in specific areas, and circumstances will be further determined by the laws and regulations of heritage management in the country where the site is located. In areas that have well-preserved sites or are protected monuments, it is more likely that non-invasive techniques such as aerial photography, field walking, and geophysical survey will be permitted before approval to undertake an invasive excavation are permitted.

Box 1. Excavation of a Subsidiary Healing Sanctuary to
the Goddess Hygieia

This is a fictitious site located in an area below mountains and about two kilometres from the sea, somewhere in the eastern Mediterranean. The site has a particular number, let us say 101 and year 2010. So it would be something like, Sanctuary to Hygieia, city/county, and country 101/2010.

A team of archaeologists from a university in northern Europe and the country in question have joined forces to undertake a further examination of a healing sanctuary to the Greek god Asclepius that was originally excavated in the 1920s. The

(continued)

idea developed when two colleagues from each university were writing papers on different elements of the excavated area and both became aware of a possible extension or separate sanctuary located next to the excavated Asclepion. When looking through previous site reports, they noticed a thoroughly recorded list of inscriptions. Fortunately, not only were the inscriptions documented in detail, but their provenance was noted, something that was not always carried out in early archaeological studies. Roughly thirty inscriptions dedicated to the goddess Hygieia were found outside the *temenos*, an enclosed sacred area, of the sanctuary of Asclepius lying randomly in a field to the west of the site. The inscriptions, mainly altar dedications, were removed and stored in the museum associated with the sanctuary. Although these inscriptions had been recorded, no archaeologist had considered what their relationship was to the Asclepion. This re-evaluation incited the archaeologists to ask whether the altars might indicate a separate sanctuary associated with the goddess Hygieia. In relation to this, they also wanted to know the dates of its use, if there were any structures associated with it, if it was a separate sanctuary, and what the boundaries of the site were.

In order to consider the questions, they organized a team of excavators that consisted of themselves as site directors, site supervisors from both universities' archaeological staff and from the universities' associated archaeological field units, and excavators who were mainly students and local volunteers. As directors, they had to decide the location of their excavation trenches. There are a number of ways they could do this. First, they examined aerial photographs of the area to see if there were visible crop marks that indicated structures, roadways, or boundaries. They also visited the site to carry out field walking to see if there was a concentration of artefacts in particular areas. Field walking involves lining people up and walking across an area of land that is divided by a measured grid. The grid helps archaeologists locate artefact concentrations. This activity is easier to do when the soil has been ploughed because the turned soil will bring artefacts to the surface of the ground. They also performed a geophysical survey to see if any anomalies appeared beneath the surface of the soil. Although there is a lot of faith placed in this method, it is far from foolproof. Sometimes features do not appear in the survey, but then show up in the excavation, and other times features appear in the geophysical survey that are non-existent in the excavation. The team also set up a series of test trenches located at regular intervals across the western area of the site to determine concentrated places of human activity. From these surveys, they were able to determine the best locations for their main excavation trenches (Fig. 1).

In this case, the aerial photographs and geophysical survey revealed a rectangular structure in the centre of what appears to be a wall surrounding the site.

(continued)

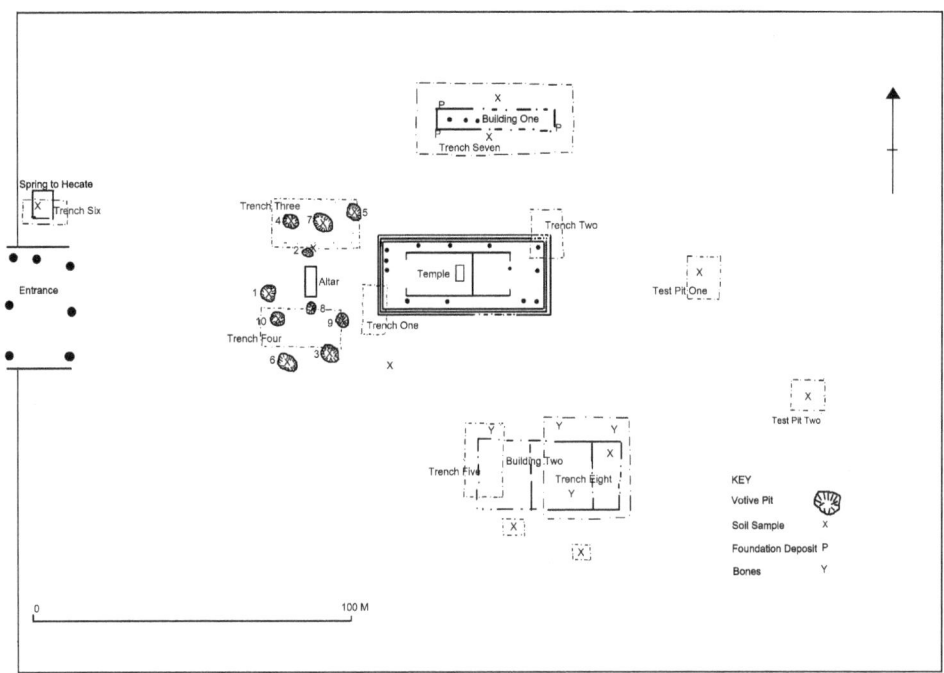

1. Invented site plan of the Healing Sanctuary of Hygieia. Drawing by the author.

The field walking and test trenches indicated most of the activity (or most of the artefacts) occurred in the northern part of the site and around the western front of the rectangular structure. From this, the team created an excavation plan that called for three seasons (years) of four weeks of excavation each. In the first year, they decided to open four trenches: one on the western end of the rectangular structure, one on its eastern end, and two where there were concentrations of pottery on the northern side of the structure. Each trench was laid out to measure 12.0 × 8.0 metres, but there is no standard size, and this is determined by the archaeologists, often in consultation with the heritage manager. In the second year, they examined the northern and southern sides of the structure, and in the third year, some possible surrounding buildings that appeared in the geophysical survey and in the test trenches. Not only were the excavations carried out by those mentioned above, but geologists and environmental specialists were also brought in to determine what the landscape and environment was like at the time of the site's use and construction.

Even when all of the above methods of preliminary testing and organization had been carried out, the archaeologists could not simply begin to dig; they had to survey the site so that it could be measured and mapped in order to pinpoint it in the local area if they wished to return to initiate further work on the site. They also set

(continued)

up a grid, laid out in square-metre measurements across the site. This helps to locate trenches and features across the area. The trenches were laid out, and each was given a particular number. They were carefully measured to make sure the angles and sides were straight. The archaeologists chose to make the trenches rectangular, but there is no standard size. Most trenches are quadrilateral.

Once the preliminary tasks were performed, the excavations began. Again, there are numerous ways to dig. Archaeologists can choose simply to trowel a site and locate artefacts in the soil, or they can sieve the soil through screens to detect smaller finds, a method that is commonly used in American archaeology and early prehistoric periods. Wet sieving can also be employed. This process entails placing soil samples in water and gently agitating the water to loosen the soil. This allows light materials such as seeds and tiny bones to float to the top of the container, while the heavier materials such as pebbles and soil sink to the bottom of the container. Seeds, particularly carbonized ones, indicate what people might have been growing and eating at the time of occupation. Small bones also might demonstrate what people were eating, or the fauna that lived in the area. Fish bones, if found on inland sites away from a major water source, can be representative of importation. In relation to the environment, the soil samples on the site in question were also examined for pollens and insect remains. This explained the plants and animals that were living in the area, and helped to reconstruct the local environment. It was determined that the area was mainly grassy with a few olive and cypress trees growing in the vicinity. To locate metal artefacts, the archaeologists would sometimes use a metal detector across the site and over spoil heaps to locate metal finds that might be missed in trowelling. When they detected metal finds in the trenches, they placed a marker over the area to warn the archaeologist that a metal find might be lurking beneath the soil. Never would an archaeologist dig straight down to find the object because this would take it out of its archaeological stratigraphic layer.

Although digging is exciting, it is not simply a treasure hunt for objects. Careful records were kept of where objects were found within a trench to help determine dates, associated artefacts, and a context. Trenches are therefore excavated stratigraphically. Often stratigraphic layers are described as a layer cake of soil that is stacked on top of one another. However, it is usually never this straightforward, and Deetz's analogy to a layer cake that has been dropped is more suitable (Fig. 2). Each strata of soil was given a context number and indicated different dates. The layers were drawn in section and as a plan which might show features (Figs. 1 and 2), photographs were taken, and all the finds from each layer were recorded and catalogued with numbers pertaining to the site, trench, and stratigraphic layer. Any feature, such as foundations, walls, pits, post-holes, column bases, or burials,

(continued)

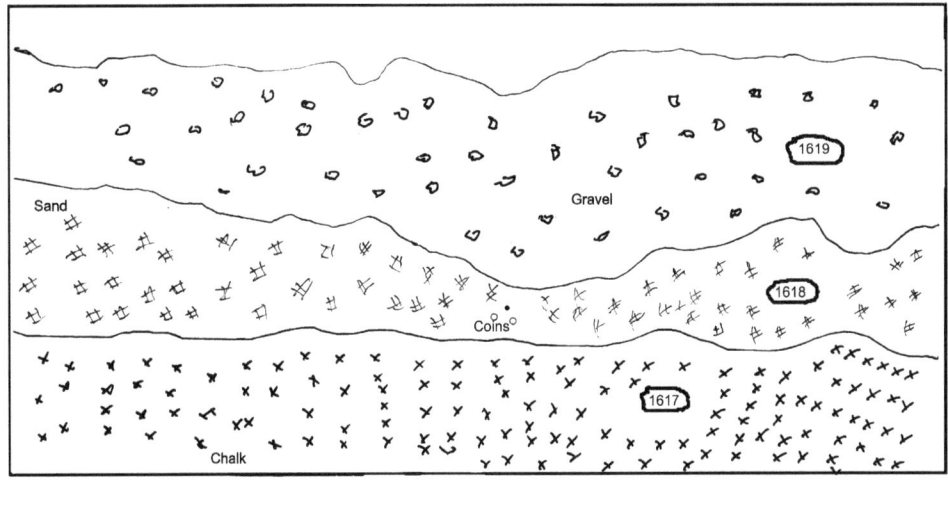

2. Invented plan of stratigraphic layers in the Sanctuary of Hygieia. Drawing by the author.

were given a separate feature number and marked for the layer(s) in which they were found.

During the periods of excavation, there were daily discussions by everyone involved with the digging about what they found. Each day, new things were revealed, producing more questions. Sometimes trenches were extended or new ones opened. At the end of the three-year period, the archaeologists identified the rectangular structure as a Roman period temple dating to the first century AD, on account of foundations, column bases, and the remains of pediments and an Ionic frieze. They also found the foundations of a wall that ran around the site, and ten pits filled with votive offerings were found, most of them close to the western side of the temple. These were found close to the foundations of a small structure thought to be the altar, located in front of the temple. There were a few structures found around the temple, but their functions were indeterminate.

After each season was over, the archaeologists cleaned and catalogued the artefacts. The soil samples taken from the site were examined for their environmental remains. A yearly report was written explaining what had happened during the excavations. Ultimately, the entire excavation was published as a site report. Depending on the scale of the site, a site report will consist of either one or two large volumes or a series of volumes dedicated to specific features and artefacts. Although each site will be published differently, there are some general rules that apply to site reports. For the most part, they will contain a section about the excavations that describe

(continued)

the trenches, the structures identified, maps, and descriptions of the different stages of development of the site over time. Sometimes these can be complicated. The remainder of the publication(s) is/are usually dedicated to small finds, which are divided into different categories and written up by a find's specialist: pottery (fine and courseware), iron objects, clay objects, copper alloy objects, coins, inscriptions, and bones (human and animal). Sometimes there is an environmental section. In theory, the objects should be cross-referenced so that it is clear what was found together. However, this is not always indicated in site reports. There will also be a discussion about what the site might have been used for and when it was occupied, but for the most part, many of the interpretations made about the objects and the site will stem from these reports. Hence, the reports are an invaluable reference for further consideration and research by other scholars.

As mentioned, some of the remains will be studied by specialists, and in certain instances, these experts will work in lab-based archaeological sciences. The soil and flotation samples taken from the site were studied in an archaeological lab under a microscope to determine the types of plants and insects that were common to the region. One of the samples was taken from inside the room (trench 8, Fig. 1), and it was found to have a lot of charred seeds, indicating a possible hearth that might have been used for cooking foods.

Although no human bones were found in the sanctuary, possibly because of restrictions placed on the association with death in ancient sanctuaries, animal bones were found and these were sent to biological anthropologists who study bones. The animal bones were examined to determine the type of animals and to see if there were signs of butchering in trenches 3, 4, 5, and 8 (Fig. 1). It was found that the animal bones located near the altar (trenches 3 and 4) were all those of sheep, and showed signs of butchering and burning. It is argued that the animals were used in ritual sacrifice and possibly butchered and cooked. The bones found in trenches 5 and 8 (Fig. 1) were different. Trenches 5 and 8 contained a building, number two. The bones found outside of the building were from rodents, which may have lived in the site, while those inside the building were a mix of chicken, cattle, and pig, all of which had signs of butchering and burning. The environmental samples from the same room of the building also indicated that the room had a hearth, most likely used for cooking.

In the same room, three complete pottery vessels were found. One had the remains of seeds and insects in it. In comparison to some medical texts, it was found that some pharmaceutical recipes contained the same seeds and insects, so it might have been that this pot held a specific remedy. The other two were studied for their residues. Animal fats were discovered in both of them, possibly indicating that they were used for cooking and/or storing animal products.

(continued)

Some of the metal scalpels found at the site had their blades attached. These were sent off to labs for use-wear analysis and to see if there were signs of blood on them, which might indicate whether they had been used on animals or humans. In the end, the cutting tools were found to have been dulled by use, and it is assumed that they were used either on humans for treatment or on animals for sacrifice. There were no signs of blood on the remaining instruments, so their use on people and/or animals cannot be indicated with any certainty.

For our site, all of the theoretical premises discussed above could be used to interpret the archaeological remains. A cultural historian would mainly be interested in dating the area and describing the site and the finds within it. They would also be concerned with noting who might have used it and to which group of people it belonged.

Although this interpretative method provides us with important information about the site, much more could be made of the remains. A processualist might wish to incorporate Middle Range Theory and make a comparison of modern groups of people. The pits of votive objects could be compared with the modern religious practice, local to the region, where votive objects were also used to see if they were deposited in comparable manners, which could indicate analogous practices. They would also be concerned about the environment and whether the structures were built in regards to the local weather conditions.

A postprocessualist would be more interested in asking questions about who worshipped at the site, how they did it, why they did it in the area, and what they would have experienced. They could take a gendered approach by asking if the votives and inscriptions were sex specific, and ask what this might indicate about the people worshipping at the sanctuary. They might take a neo-Marxist approach and ask if there is evidence for a social hierarchy in relation to the worshippers and the priests, or they may wish to understand specific depositional practices of objects to see how people felt about specific practices related to healing. Another aspect that archaeologists may wish to consider is how this material can be presented to the public. They decided that this should be re-created, as it was in the second century AD, because this seemed to be the period when it was most active. However, by choosing to reconstruct the site at this time, later period structures were left incomplete. Therefore, it must be realized that when people visit sites, they are visiting them in accordance with the choices of the museum curators, heritage managers, and archaeologists. The question that always needs to be addressed is why it is re-created to a particular period. In the case of object display, again the question is why there are certain items on display and why others are in the museum store or site archive.

2.5 CONCLUSION

For historians of medicine, the excavation will be less important than the objects that survive from them. However, it is important to understand how materials are acquired and catalogued, especially if site reports are consulted. The various methods of interpretations mentioned in this chapter will be explained further in the following chapters when the different categories of artefacts and structures are discussed.

CONSIDERATION QUESTIONS

1. Consider whether there are similarities between the development of medical historical theoretical and methodological approaches with some of the archaeological approaches to theory and practice mentioned in this chapter. Do you think there are reasons why this might or might not be the case?

2. Do you think some of the basic archaeological theories mentioned could also be applied to textual sources? Why or why not?

FURTHER READING

Barker, P. 1986. *Understanding Archaeological Excavations*. London: B. T. Batsford.
  2002. *Techniques of Archaeological Excavation*. London: Routledge.
Binford, L. R. 1972. *An Archaeological Perspective*. New York: Seminar Press.
Bintliff, J., and M. Pearce, eds. 2011. *The Death of Archaeological Theory*. Oxford: Oxbow Books.
Deetz, J. 1996 (rev. ed.). *In Small Things Forgotten: The Archaeology of Early American Life*. New York: Anchor, Doubleday.
Hodder, I. 1982. *The Present Past: An Introduction to Anthropology for Archaeologists*. London: B. T. Batsford.
  1996. *Theory and Practice in Archaeology*. London: Routledge.
  2007 (7th ed.). *The Archaeological Process: An Introduction*. Oxford: Blackwell.
Hodder, I., and S. Hutson 2003 (3rd ed.). *Reading the Past: Current Approaches to Interpretation in Archaeology*. Cambridge: Cambridge University Press.
Hodder, I., and R. Pruecel, eds. 1996. *Contemporary Archaeology in Theory*. Oxford: Blackwell.
Johnson, M. 2009 (2nd ed.). *Archaeological Theory an Introduction*. Oxford: Blackwell.
Praetzellis, A. 2003. *Dug to Death: A Tale of Archaeological Method and Mayhem*. New York: Altamira Press.
  2011 (rev. ed.). *Death by Theory: A Tale of Mystery and Archaeological Theory*. New York: Altamira Press.
Renfrew, C., and P. Bahn 2005. *Archaeology: The Key Concepts*. London: Routledge.
Shanks, M., and C. Tilley 1987. *Social Theory in Archaeology*. Cambridge: Polity Press.
  1992. *Reconstructing Archaeology, Theory and Practice*. London: Routledge.
Trigger, B. 2006 (2nd ed.). *A History of Archaeological Thought*. Cambridge: Cambridge University Press.

CHAPTER 3

TEXT AS MATERIAL CULTURE

3.1 INTRODUCTION

Emily Vermeule, a distinguished Bronze Age archaeologist, was elected president of the American Philological Association (APA) in 1995, a professional organization dedicated to the study of Greek and Latin. In her presidential address, she said the APA "perpetrated a cosmic joke in electing a Bronze Age archaeologist as their president" (1996: 1). In her speech, she attempted to reconcile two disciplines she had found to be at odds with one another throughout her long career as an archaeologist – archaeology and the study of ancient literature. The uneasy division she referred to is not exclusive to classical archaeology and has been the subject of considerable discussion by archaeologists who work with both textual sources and material remains (e.g. Baker 2002a: 16–19; Christie 2011: 3–4; Deetz 1977, 1996; Galloway 2006; Hicks and Beaudry 2006; Moreland 2007; Sauer 2004; Tarlow 1999). Numerous explanations have been given to explain why this division exists, some of which were briefly mentioned in Chapter 1 of this book. Vermeule's professional experience led her to conclude that those who dig, or work with dirt, are considered to be part of the mechanical arts, while those who work with words are in the field of the liberal arts. She concluded that words appear to be more highly prized in academic circles, and on a basic level, this is possibly because they are "cleaner than the dirt" (1996: 2). Her delivery was not intended to be a comprehensive account of the academic disparities. Rather, she introduced some concerns pertaining to how scholars from different areas of study react to subjects outside of their own fields of expertise. She concluded that one of the main difficulties that stems from this division is a lack of interdisciplinary discussion and awareness of other subjects, which, to reiterate, is the central problem this book addresses.

In order to make the subject of archaeology relevant to scholars outside of the discipline, this chapter applies archaeological questions to the source of evidence most commonly used by medical historians – texts. In the previous chapters, we saw how texts often omit important information about everyday social practices. In this chapter, we will see how texts have material properties and how these properties can be just as significant as the words written on them. We will see how the act of writing and the words themselves play a distinctive role in procedures and rituals relating to healing and attempts to bring about illness. Examinations extending beyond translations, which consider how texts were intended to be read, manufactured, displayed, and stored, can enhance our awareness of how social rules regarding the transmission of medical practices and knowledge were conveyed to different groups of people. Indeed, texts are both tangibly and intangibly culturally manipulated objects. Tangibly, they are written on particular materials in certain handwriting styles that are temporally and regionally specific. Intangibly, their meaning is determined by their grammatical structure (Deetz 1967: 83–96; 1977: 24–5; Galloway 2006: 43–4).

This chapter is divided into five sections. In the first section, an explanation is given about why archaeological sources are useful to historical studies. The second accounts for the scholarly debates that have taken place between historians and archaeologists. This discussion will expand upon some of the issues mentioned in Chapter 1 in order to show how the immediate context of scholarship requires more interdisciplinary dialogue. The emphasis on texts as material remains, nonetheless, should not be understood to be saying that it is only those who examine texts who are dismissive of other disciplines. This is definitely not the case. Material cultural specialists can also be indifferent to textual sources. Thus, the third part of this chapter is devoted to introducing archaeologists, who may be unfamiliar with how to use translations in their work, to problems with textual translation. The fourth section then introduces the documentary evidence examined by medical historians. The aims here are to familiarize archaeologists with the various types of textual remains that are available for study and to demonstrate how these remains can be interpreted from an archaeological perspective. The chapter will conclude with an examination of how the act of writing and the text itself can take on "non-utilitarian" functions that serve purposes beyond conventional conceptions of texts as providing, for example, a historical account or philosophical argument.

3.2 THE NEED TO STUDY MATERIAL REMAINS

The combined use of textual and archaeological remains should be considered an asset to historical scholarship. The two types of evidence cannot only

fill gaps where there is little or no existing evidence in one source of information. When both sources of information are available, they can be compared
to see if the same interpretation or "story" is plausible. As we have already
seen to some extent, in some instances, the archaeological remains and historical evidence complement each other, and in others they contradict one
another. This latter point is especially pertinent because the archaeological
evidence can show where an historical text might be biased or exaggerated
in its account. In addition, if the archaeological remains account for everyday practices often omitted from texts, they can "give a voice" to the "silent
majority" in the past who did not leave us written accounts.

3.3 INTERDISCIPLINARY APPROACHES TO HISTORICAL
PERIOD ARCHAEOLOGY

The term historical archaeology, like archaeology, does not have a universal
definition. Most scholars who classify themselves as historical archaeologists
tend to work on remains that date from the fifteenth century to the present
(Hicks and Beaudry 2006: 1). Others argue that the term can be applied to
any society with written records (Moreland 2007). Both definitions are problematic: the former for ignoring earlier periods with writing, and the latter
because, in some instances, a society with writing did co-exist with another
which had no written record. Put simply, this means that both prehistoric
and historic societies existed alongside one another. When this happened,
records about the people living in non-literate societies were made by those
living in literate groups. For instance, we see this in the Hippocratic text of
Airs Waters Places (17–22) where the writer described the lifestyle and health
of the Scythians. This is referred to as an ethnohistorical or sometimes protohistorical period because one society writes about another in a similar vein
to modern anthropological examinations of indigenous people (Praetzellis
2003: 72–4).

Since there is abundant textual evidence available from the ancient world,
it would seem appropriate to place it under the remit of historical archaeology. Yet, classical archaeology is classified as a separate subdivision from
other areas of archaeology, indicated by the fact it is often taught in classics
departments rather than in anthropology or archaeology departments, particularly in North America (see Chapter 4). In spite of this, it shares the same
fundamental problems of archaeological interpretation and historiography
with historical and protohistorical (ethnohistorical) archaeologists (Sauer
2004). At the same time, classical archaeology could also be considered ethnohistorical because there are written Greek and Roman accounts of people

from places where no indigenous writing survives. See, for example, the Hippocratic text just mentioned along with the work of other writers – that is, Herodotus' (4.61–81) description of the Scythians and the Roman writer Tacitus' account of the Germans in his *Germania*.

Due to the variant manners in which archaeological sub-disciplines can be defined, it is arguable that they are too restrictive, forcing scholars to justify why their work fits into one or more of these categories. Since the categories have overlapping aspects, rather than trying to force a topic into one classification, it would seem more beneficial for the archaeologist dealing with various problems of interpretation to talk to another scholar who has encountered similar difficulties. However one may define "historical" and "classical archaeology", the one feature that brings sub-disciplines together is the problem of understanding both textual and material remains. And these, of course, are not possessed exclusively by any one discipline. Texts and material remains are available to any archaeologist or historian who has a question about them.

3.3.1 Relationship between History and Archaeology

Another variation of the problem of boundaries exists between distinctly demarcated subjects. Scholars will sometimes have to justify the existence of their discipline to others outside their discipline. Moreland (2007: 13–16) argues that those who work with material remains are often placed in a position where they have to defend their subject in response to misunderstandings about archaeology by scholars who focus on texts. Part of the problem, according to Moreland, stems from the archaeologists themselves. They have managed to make their discipline seem less important than textual histories through the manner in which they promote the subject. Rather than arguing that material culture is informative about social rules or explaining how archaeologists reach their conclusions, archaeologists will often defend their position by stating that archaeology is important where no texts exist. Yet, when there is a text, they tend not to note the necessity for studying the material remains in conjunction with written evidence (2007: 16–21). Consequently, artefacts become the proverbial "handmaiden to history". This means that physical remains are only deemed useful for supporting historical texts, rather than being seen as a valid form of evidence in their own right.

To corroborate his view, Moreland (2007: 54–76) considered how and when the idea developed that the text is a more legitimate form of information to study than material remains. He observed that texts began to take precedence over spoken words in the seventeenth century, notably after the invention of the printing press. Prior to this, there was a greater emphasis on oral tradition. Often what was written was either a record of a speech or something intended to be read aloud. This is possibly because reading was not an integral skill for many people to have needed in the past, especially since a majority of books were copied and held in monasteries and were not readily available for general consultation. Hence, the written word was not an expedient form of communication in many instances, and because of this, messages were passed on through verbal and bodily communication, as well as through artistic representations and material remains. This also means that the archaeological record may be in fact richer in terms of variety of evidence and more informative about life in the past.

3.3.2 The Promotion of Interdisciplinary Approaches

There have been attempts by archaeologists to bring together the different disciplines through conference discussions and edited volumes. In 1995, Small edited a book that considered the relationship between historians and archaeologists of the Greco-Roman world (see especially Dyson, Ober, and Small's papers 1995). In terms of conferences, I co-organized a session with A. Gardner at the Theoretical Archaeology Group (TAG) conference in 2000 on *Material Histories and Textual Archaeologies*. A year later, the theme was raised again at TAG by E. Sauer who subsequently published the proceedings of the session (2004). In November 2011, a conference was organized by D. Stewart entitled *Crossing the Divide: Archaeology and Ancient History* at Leicester University, England. Interestingly, the same themes were broached in these conferences and the edited volumes: consideration of the combined use of materials, text as a form of material culture, and the relationship between different fields of scholarship. In spite of the interesting discussion they generated, the participants were, for the most part, archaeologists who already used an interdisciplinary approach in their work. Conversely, some historians have made initial calls for interdisciplinary discussion between historians and archaeologists. See, for instance, a recent edited collection concerned with the use of material remains in historical studies for the eighteenth, nineteenth, and twentieth centuries (Harvey 2009) and Laurence's (2012) *Roman Archaeology for Historians*, which is a short history of the field of Roman archaeology that includes discussions of recent scholarly debates, rather than an introduction to archaeological methods. The attempts to bridge the gap between fields of study are encouraging because they demonstrate the willingness to understand methods and materials commonly limited to particular disciplines. Despite this dialogue, there remains much work to be done.

As one would expect, counterarguments have been put forth in order to maintain disciplinary boundaries. The main reason involves a concern over the lack of necessary training to bridge one or more disciplines. Indeed, scholars trained in one discipline may lack the necessary tuition to study another discipline (Rankov 2004: 55). In some cases, the rationale behind this is evident. For instance, there are times when historians attempt to use archaeological material in their studies or make comments about it, but do not demonstrate an understanding of critical archaeological methodologies (e.g. Green 2004; Salazar 2000: 230). Conversely, lack of expertise is also apparent with archaeologists who know little about referencing and using ancient textual sources, or worse still, what is said in the texts can be taken uncritically at face value (e.g. Roberts and Manchester 2005). Nonetheless, these problems should not be seen as insurmountable or as reasons to break off from a professional responsibility to understand evidence in other interpretive and explanatory contexts. Obtaining a solid background to other disciplines is feasible, and, in fact, the problems mentioned above demonstrate that a better understanding is taking place, albeit initially in the form of criticism.

There are also a number of archaeologists and philologists who have training outside of their fields. Some are equally adept at translating historical texts and interpreting material remains. While some may be stronger in one area than another, they tend to be familiar enough with both fields to make reasonable judgements about the types of materials with which they are working.

3.4 WORKING WITH TEXTS

A brief comment is made here for archaeologists who are interested in using texts, but may not be proficient in language training. There are numerous translations of ancient sources, but they are not all of equal value for academic purposes. Some may be intended for more general use, and there may be some liberties taken with the translation when the original language is not provided. On a practical level, these translations do not always provide book, chapter, and line numbers used in academic editions of ancient texts. Or, if they do, the numbers may differ. This means it will be difficult to check the translated text against the original language. Popular versions of texts rarely have a commentary that explains how the document has come down to us through time, which manuscripts were used in reproducing the text, and where the different manuscripts have textual variations. Even when critical commentaries and academic translations are incorporated, the reader must always keep in mind that the translations will vary depending on the bias of the translator. Although they may be trying to translate as true to the original text as possible, there will be choices they have to make about the meanings of particular words, especially if the context is unclear. In such instances, a meaning unintended by the original author may be given by the translator.

Another problem that can contribute to changes in the original meaning of the text is an expectation that published translations should "read well" in English. In Sachs' introduction to his translation of Aristotle's *Metaphysics*, he makes it clear that his translation will read rather roughly in places because he is attempting to capture the essence of Aristotle's words and phrases. He notes that

> From the point of view of a classicist, a good English translation of a classical author is one that finds, for every word or phrase in the original, some equivalent expression that reads smoothly in our language. This may be good practice with some kinds of writing, but philosophical meanings cannot be captured in habitual uses of language. The point of view of a professional philosopher may, however, pay too much heed to the linguistic choices that have become habitual in modern philosophy and in the secondary literature, at the expense of faithfulness to the original. (2002: xxxv)

This problem can be exacerbated if the original text cannot be referred to in order to check the translation. I have found in my own work that historians may read a meaning into a text that is actually not clear in the original language. Even what appears to be very minor can have significant consequences for an argument. For example, a statement about the emperor Severus Alexander is often used as confirmation that the sick and wounded soldiers were kept in separate quarters from the healthy soldiers (*S. H. A. Severus Alexander* 47. 2). It is stated that when the emperor was on campaign, he visited the sick in their tents: *"aegrotantes ipse visitavit per tentoria milites"*. Since the writer uses the plural for tents (*tentoria*), it is difficult to determine if the soldiers were simply placed in their regular tents, or if a group of tents was placed together for the hospital. To our modern eye, these questions are difficult to ascertain from the statement. A number of readings are possible. Yet, at the time this was written, this statement might have been clearly understood by those who read it.

Scholars must also consider how texts are transmitted through time, as the manner of their survival also affects how they are translated. A Greek Hippocratic text, for example, would be replicated for libraries and perhaps private collections over an extended period of time. During the Byzantine period, many classical Greek manuscripts were copied by monks for monastery

libraries, some of which continued to be reproduced in their original languages while others were translated into vernacular languages. Over time,
some texts were translated into Hebrew and Arabic and eventually translated
back into Latin or Greek. Since they were duplicated and translated, perhaps many times, mistakes occurred. Some versions of texts have different
words or phrases added to them; some texts are known to have existed but
have been lost; and, in some instances, the translators or copyists might have
added their own ideas to the document, altering the meaning of the original
version. Sometimes texts thought to have been lost or never known to have
existed are found in old monastery libraries (see Reynolds and Wilson 1978
for a full discussion). Like artefacts, newly found texts can change understandings of older scholarly interpretations.

Therefore, archaeologists interested in using texts should find critical
editions of translations that explain the condition of the work and compare
differences in the various surviving manuscripts. Even if the original language
is not known to the scholar, it will be possible to see where the text is corrupt
or if there are alternative translations, allowing for a more investigative use
of the translations that might otherwise be missed if a general translation is
employed.

3.5 TEXTUAL SOURCES AS MATERIAL CULTURE

Besides the erudite medical and philosophical texts of authors such as Galen,
Rufus of Ephesus, and the Hippocratic writers, medical historians are fortunate to have many other types of textual remains at their disposal that survive from the Greco-Roman period: papyri fragments, lead curse tablets, wax
and wood tablets, inscriptions, coins, and collyrium stamps. There existed
entire industries related to the manufacture of some of these documents, be
it for personal or public use. Although translating them is often illuminating,
studying them for their archaeological properties can enlighten us about the
fabrication of the texts and the manner in which they were intended to be
viewed, transported, used, and stored. The fabric can tell us about the technologies of the time, the trade in materials, and even the possible social and/
or monetary value of the texts. Inscribed objects also required specific writing tools such as inks, metals, paints, and writing and carving implements.
So, other concerns can be addressed such as asking where these materials
were processed, copied, stored, read, and displayed, and where libraries or
structure were located. For a modern example, one need only think about
how modern technologies are changing the way we access and read books,
ancient and medieval manuscripts, and journal articles. The Internet and

computer technology allow us to access texts at the press of a button that might not be in our libraries. By comparing the subjects written on the documents with their archaeological properties, it may be possible to see if social rules existed about whether texts containing certain types of information had to be inscribed on specific materials and/or treated in particular manners. Such a comparison helps to provide deeper insights into the manner in which people thought about written documents associated with healing in the past.

3.5.1 Who Studies These Textual Remains?

The textual sources mentioned above are examined by different types of scholars, which has led to fragmented specialisms within the fields of Greek and Latin literature. Although there may seem to be no logical reason why certain materials have become the concern for specific specialists, such as ostraca being studied by papyrologists, this specialization developed because there are vast amounts of materials that require different conventions of translation. Consider how names normally painted on Greek vases are the concern of art historians who catalogue and describe images on pottery. Yet, words carved or stamped into large clay vessels are studied and catalogued by epigraphers, who are mainly responsible for the study of inscriptions on marble, stone, bronze, or lead. Anything written in ink usually falls under the remit of the papyrologist, such as papyri, ostraca, and wooden tablets. Numismatists study the inscriptions on coins (Bodel 2001: 2–5).

A number of problems must be negotiated when working with original texts of these sorts. First, they can be written in local dialects and/or have words borrowed from regional languages, which are sometimes untranslatable. Abbreviations are also used, particularly on epigraphic remains and coins, which may not always be interpreted correctly. Graphic styles are temporally and regionally specific, and in some cases may appear to be indecipherable; so many of the experts will have training in palaeography, the study of ancient handwriting. These textual and stylistic differences arose from various local customs, politics, and materials being made available at different times and places (Bodel 2001: 6–13).

3.5.2 Readership

When examining all forms of written remains, it is always essential to ask who the intended readership was. This can often be determined through the writing style and manner of presentation. Ancient medical texts, for example, were sometimes intended for students and at other times doctors. What of the readership for inscriptions on public monuments? No literacy statistics exist for the ancient world, though it is generally believed that a majority of people were illiterate (Harris cited in Bodel 2001: 15–16). Thus, Bodel (2001: 16), as well as others, have asked what the role of public texts was if most of the public was unable to read them.

From an archaeological perspective, this matter can be addressed by considering the provenance of the texts, which includes noting their location in terms of how and where they were intended to be viewed. For example, an inscription on a public building might have been an indicator of the building's importance. Even if a passer-by could not read the words, the lettering on it could have symbolized its significance. In another instance, copies of laws and decrees that were read aloud were positioned in general view as a reminder of the event at which they were announced. Its significance, therefore, could be recalled in public memory. This could also apply to religious altars and funerary monuments. Alternatively, if texts were stored in private homes or libraries, then the readership would have been smaller, and perhaps the documents would have been more specialized. In such instances, the location indicates the activities that might have occurred in the space, such as reading and studying, undertaken by a specific group of people. Therefore, the structure in which the texts were found, if they exist, can be examined to see what the studying and learning environments might have been like in the ancient world.

There has been much excitement with the recent discovery of a previously lost work by Galen entitled *On Consolation from Grief* (*Peri Alupēsias*). The work is a letter from Galen explaining the loss of his medical books, drugs, and medical instruments that were stored in a warehouse in Rome that caught fire (Nicholls 2010, 2011; Nutton 2009; Tucci 2008). In this letter, he lists the books that were in his private collection and how libraries were run. It seems that books were written in libraries, and this text is a wonderful resource for understanding how doctors and scholars studied and consulted manuscripts in the Roman world.

3.5.3 Dating and Demography

Fundamentally, textual remains can be a useful resource in archaeology for ascertaining the dates of objects and sites. Dates of important events were usually inscribed on public monuments. For materials which do not have such an inscription, a date can still be established from the style of writing and the use of particular words and phrases that were common at certain times in the past (Keppie 1991: 28–9). However, even when a date is given, it cannot be taken for granted that the date is accurate. This is because sometimes a new monument makes use of older elements. For instance, the arch of Constantine in Rome has relief sculptures attached to it that originally formed parts of earlier monuments (Ramage and Ramage 2000: 226). Sometimes the original commemoration is left on a newer version of a monument or structure. The Pantheon in Rome that survives today was reconstructed during Hadrian's reign. Hadrian replaced the original structure commissioned by Agrippa a century earlier. However, he left Agrippa's commemoration on it (Ramage and Ramage 2000: 226).

Coins that have images of kings and emperors are useful for dating because they would have been minted during the period of their respective rulership. When these are found with a set of objects in a particular stratigraphic layer (Fig. 2), they can be used to date the artefacts found within the same layer. Let us say we have a coin from the reign of Caracalla with the image of Asclepius on it (Penn 1994: 41, fig. 28). We know that Caracalla reigned from AD 198–217, so the coin had to be issued within this period of time. This means that the coin could not have been used, deposited, or dropped before AD 198. Thus, anything below the layer in which the coin was found is designated as "the time before which" or *terminus ante quem* (TAQ). Yet, since the coins were not only used during his reign and could be in use for a couple of hundred years after the date, anything found in the same stratigraphic layers and those above it will date to the period in which the coin was minted or after it. This in archaeology is known as "TPQ" or *terminus post quem* ("the time after which").

Grave steles that give a person's age at the time of their death are sometimes used to establish the average age of mortality in particular regions. Demographic information of this sort has been referred to in some historical studies, but a word of caution needs to be given about the kind of evidence bearing inscriptions designating age. Revel (2005) has pointed out that there are regional differences in commemorating the Roman dead, so there will not be a representative sample of some groups of people, such as women or children. Along with this, she notes that ages inscribed on Roman epitaphs were often rounded to numbers ending in zero or five, so an accurate age might not be known.

3.5.4 Papyrus and Parchment

Medical texts written by the likes of Galen and Diocles, for example, would originally have been written on papyrus or parchment in the form of book rolls. Two-thirds of the medical texts that have been found on papyrus are from the *Hippocratic Corpus* and the many works of Galen (Jones 2009: 355). Nonetheless, it is not simply the erudite literature that can be used to provide evidence about ancient medicine. Papyri fragments of letters written to families and doctors explaining illnesses and treatments have been recovered. Greco-Roman magical papyri were sometimes used to invoke a cure for a disease or to cause someone to become ill as a form of revenge. Sometimes records of people's health were recorded on official documents. For example, there is a discharge paper for a man who had weak eyesight due to a cataract (*P.Oxy* 39; Davies 1969a: 211; Watson 1969: 41). There is a letter from a soldier to his father apologizing for not writing because his entire unit had come down with food poisoning from rancid fish. The letter also indicates he had been cared for by his friends (*P.Mich* 478). A fragment exists of an order form for a blanket to be sent to the military *valetudinarium* in Cappadocia (*BGU* 1564=Sp 395, papyrus Egypt 138; Campbell 1994: 239), which explains that the blanket had to be made a certain size. All of these seemingly minor texts tell us something about medical practices in the past. We learn that people could be discharged from their duties on account of their physical condition, soldiers helped each other when ill, and that a *valetudinarium* existed and supplies were ordered for it.

Papyrus was made from the *Cyperus Papyrus L.* plant that was cultivated in Egypt and possibly Syria and Mesopotamia (Bülow-Jacobsen 2009: 5). Pliny (*HN* 13.23–5, 74–82) explains that papyrus paper was made by weaving together strands of papyrus; it was moistened with water and mud from the Nile to glue it, and then it was pressed on a flat board. Experiments have been made to attempt to recreate the process described by Pliny, but the results were not consistent with the papyri found in the archaeological record. So it seems that another process might have been employed (Bülow-Jacobsen 2009: 5–10). It can, however, be ascertained that a roll of papyrus most likely consisted of twenty individual sheets of papyrus that were placed together, with the left edge of one sheet lying on top of the right edge of another. Papyrus was then rolled around a wooden stick to form a roll. These were then sold, and the papyrus could be cut off the roll in order to be used as a paper supply for a variety of documents, or the roll could be left intact for an entire book or part of a book, depending on its length.

In the same discussion, Pliny (*HN* 13.23.76) also explained that there were various grades of papyrus, one of which was called *amphitheatricae* named after the place where it was manufactured. This name is thought to refer to the amphitheatre of Alexandria. If this were the case, it is a small amount of evidence that suggests variant uses for particular buildings often thought to have had a single function (something discussed in Chapter 6).

Since papyrus was only grown and processed in a small region of the Greco-Roman world, it was not a readily available resource in most places. It had to be transported to other regions as both a supply of writing materials or as finished texts. The material would have had both an economic and social value attributed to it in relation to its rarity, its scholarly content, and the distance of travel. Concerning travel, what contributed to the cost was the fact that transportation was not simple. Papyri and books were moved via the sea on cargo ships and by wagons on roads. But both methods had their distinct perils and drawbacks.

Shipping was seasonal due to the likelihood of rough seas in the winter. Even in summer, the winds and sea conditions are changeable, which may have caused delays in deliveries or, even worse, caused the ship to sink with its cargo on board. Transportation by road, therefore, might seem to have been a safer option. Although there was a substantial road system in the Greco-Roman world, travel still took time. The more remote areas were difficult to access. Road travel could also be hindered by a lack of repair, poor weather, or thieves. Thus, when there was no papyrus available, other writing materials had to be employed, such as parchment.

Parchment, initially named *pergamena* after the city of Pergamum from which it originated, was apparently invented on account of a competition for the best library between King Ptolemy V Epiphanes (205–180 BC) in Alexandria and Eumenes II (197–159 BC) of Pergamum (Pliny, *HN* 13.21.70). In order to win the competition, Ptolemy apparently prohibited the exportation of papyrus from Egypt; Eumenes was forced to find another material on which books could be written for his library. At his disposal were the skins of calves, sheep, and goats. The first part of the process in preparing the hides for writing materials was to clean them and scrape them free of hair. When they were moist, they were stretched, and while they were drying, they were treated with alum and chalk. The problem with parchment is that it required the skin of an entire animal to make a double folio page (Bülow-Jacobsen 2009: 11). However, the skins could well have been a by-product of butchering and so might have been readily available in certain places and times of the year. Since a special plant was not required, it could be crafted in more locations throughout the Greco-Roman world, which could mean that there were fewer shipping problems. Yet, the amount of material needed to complete a book would have increased the expense. Therefore, both materials were likely to have been used for important documents, rather than for general purposes, or those deemed to be important by the scholars and people living at the time. How use would have been determined is, of course, dependent on the region. The abundance of papyri in Egypt may have meant a more liberal use of writing materials when documenting.

Papyri fragments and book rolls are some of the most valuable sources for ancient texts, and these are always obtained from archaeological excavations. Since papyrus is made from natural materials, it needs the correct conditions to ensure its survival; a hot, dry climate such as Egypt is ideal. Two places in Egypt in particular have yielded high numbers of papyri documents: Oxyrhynchus and Mons Claudeanus (Cuvigny 2009: 38–42).

In the late nineteenth and early twentieth centuries, when it became apparent that ancient texts survived in these places, archaeologists formed expeditions to retrieve the objects. The hunts for papyri led to the destruction of some archaeological sites. Associated artefacts and the exact provenance of the documents usually went unrecorded. However, for those that do have a noted provenance, they tend to be found in places for waste disposal, which was particularly common at Oxyrhynchus. Sometimes it was determined that they had been reused for cartonnage, or the wraps and stuffing placed around mummies. This practice became more customary after the third century BC. In particular, outdated administrative documents and fragments of ancient literature seemed to be used in this derivative way. As will be discussed below, it is also possible that the actual writing on the documents, not the meaning of the text, was deemed to be important for ritual purposes, and this could explain why written materials were used for wrapping the dead.

In some instances, the papyrus was found in structures such as homes and record offices, though this tends to be rare in comparison to those found in the rubbish heaps (Cuvigny 2009: 45–6). According to Cuvigny (2009: 50–3), the archaeological work in rubbish heaps is unrewarding because there are a number of artefacts mixed together without a proper stratigraphy, making dating difficult. Yet, problems of stratigraphy aside, rubbish heaps provide a wealth of archaeological data. For example, it can be asked what types of items could be included in refuse dumps. Had the objects lost their importance by simply being out of date, or were people no longer interested in reading older texts? Perhaps multiple copies of certain documents existed, and the conditions of some were better than those that had been discarded or reused. The depositional practice of these objects would be of interest to see if the users were expected to deposit the texts in certain areas. Such patterns could possibly indicate social rules of some kind. It could be questioned whether letters were stored in particular places of the home, or if there were rooms in record offices that were set aside for the storage of public documents, or in the cases of magical papyri whether placement in certain locations helped in the efficacy of the spell.

The book roll was commonly used until Late Antiquity for "academic texts", including medical treatises. With the rise of Christianity in Late

Antiquity, a change occurred when the codex shape began to be used more frequently and eventually replaced the book roll. An argument put forth for this change in preference is that the codex was used by Christian writers. The scroll was associated with a literate pagan world interested in philosophical thought, while the codex, a design similar to the modern book, was generally used for record keeping, was simple, and represented more humble pursuits. Ultimately, this style became predominant and developed into the books with which we are familiar (Bülow-Jacobsen 2009: 24). Interestingly, Galen mentions that he had two codicies that were lost in the fire of AD 192. They were both lists of drug recipes, and it may be that they were notes collected together over an extended period of time and then pulled together. It would be easier to make notes on a codex than carry around a roll of papyrus or loose papyri leaves. Nicholls surmises that these might have had blank pages for Galen to add his own notes. Unlike the *volumen* (book roll), these two manuscripts were meant to be used as a reference source, not read from one end of the scroll to the other (Nicholls 2010: 383–6).

3.5.5 Wood

Because parchment and papyri were time-consuming, expensive to make, and difficult to transport, there might have been places where the importation or production of these materials was rare and not thought to have been necessary, particularly in areas with high illiteracy rates. In cases where only a few people required materials for the purposes of writing letters or for keeping records, other materials, such as wood and bark, were used. Examples of this occur at the Roman auxiliary fort of Vindolanda, located on the Stanegate Road, about a mile south of Hadrian's Wall in northern Britain. Trees were a common resource in most regions of the Greco-Roman world and provided a readily available writing material at less expense and time to manufacture than book rolls. It was, however, only preferred for short documents. Generally, a lot of ink was required for writing on wood, and, as one would suspect, it was not as malleable as papyrus or parchment.

There were two manners in which wood was used for written documents. One was as the backing for wax tablets. In this instance, a quadrilateral board had its centre scraped out, leaving four raised edges around a shallower "central well" which was filled with beeswax. The wax was written on with a stylus made of wood, bone, or copper alloy. It was usual for the stylus to have a spatula on one of its ends which could be heated for melting and smoothing the words that had been written on the wax (Bülow-Jacobsen 2009: 11). One can speculate that doctors could have used wax tablets if they were keeping medical notes about their patients, and then transferred these to other materials if they found it necessary to keep a permanent record of certain cases. Perhaps Galen did this as well, in light of his comments about codices.

The second use for wood involved writing on it directly. Thick pieces of wooden planking could be used as signs, funerary monuments, and public notices in the same manner as more permanent bronze and stone inscriptions. These were painted white and then written on with a dark ink. The white background made the lettering more visible, and inscribing the wood was less costly and time-consuming than working with permanent materials such as stone or bronze.

Thinner pieces of wood or bark were utilized as paper. There were two standardized formats for writing on the material that were dependent upon the type of document being written. The terminology may be a bit confusing here. Letters used the *landscape format* while accounts used the *letter format*. If the document was a letter, the wood was positioned in the *landscape format* (longest sides on the top and bottom and parallel to the grain of wood). This was divided into two columns, marked by a lightly scored centre. When the letter was completed, it was folded down the scored middle, and it was sealed with drawstrings. On the other hand, accounts were written in *letter format* (shorter sides on the top and bottom perpendicular to the grain of wood). If the list did not fit on one sheet of "paper", then several pieces were tied together in a concertina fashion (Bülow-Jacobsen 2009: 12–14).

The Roman auxiliary fort of Vindolanda has yielded a large collection of wooden documents consisting of military records, correspondence between soldiers and their families, and the commanding officers' wives, who were living at military sites along the frontier. They are a remarkable source of information that offer us insights into life in a military environment, as well as some medical information. Included in one of the daily military reports is a reference to health and illness. It explains who was absent from the camp and those who were unfit for duty (Inv. No. 88/841 period I dital; Bowman and Thomas 1991: 62, 66; 1994: 93–4, 98). Fifteen men were recorded as sick (*aegri*), six were listed as wounded (*vulnerati*), and ten as having eye problems (*lippientes*) (Bowman and Thomas 1991: 66–9; 1994: 93–4).

Another report is a fragmentary list that mentions 343 men who were associated with the workshop (*fabrica*), of whom twelve were shoemakers. The report then lists builders for the bathhouse; the word *valetudinarium* (hospital) follows, but there are no surviving words around it that indicate why it was mentioned. The document continues with other references to positions associated with the *fabrica* (Bowman and Thomas 1994: 155). It is possible that the word *valetudinarium* was associated with those who built it, worked in it, or made tools for it, such as medical instruments. It cannot even be determined from this whether the *valetudinarium* was a separate building or an area within another building. Without more information, we can only say that it provides an interesting link to the *fabrica*.

A third letter is fragmentary, but has an address to *Vitali seplasiario* (Bowman, Thomas, and Tomlin 2011: 125–7, no. 877). A *seplasiarius* was a person who dealt in unguents, so it is possible that there was someone stationed in Vindolanda who was responsible for ordering and possibly making ointments. Salves are recommended for all sorts of medical treatments in ancient texts, and it is likely that those living in and around the forts kept salves, perfumes, and other medicinal mixtures for personal use. We do not know if this person was of military rank or a civilian living in the region of the fort.

These documents, unlike papyri, survive because of the waterlogged conditions of the site. Some were found in the west ditch of the fort, others in wooden structures located in the *praetorium* of the camp near its south gate, and still others in structures just beyond the gate (Bowman and Thomas 1974: 4–20; 1991; 1994: 18). For the tablets found in buildings, they were located amongst eighteen inches of flooring that consisted of cut bracken, straw, gorse pods, heather, twigs, oyster shell, pottery, leather, ropes, animal bones, and human and animal dung. This flooring was compressed and could not be excavated with a trowel because troweling would destroy the documents. It was decided to use an alternative method of excavation to obtain as many tablets as possible. The flooring was, therefore, cut out of the ground in large chunks, like peat, and taken into a lab where each layer was carefully peeled away from the other. Some were held together so tightly that they could not be separated. So these were placed in water and moistened in order that the documents could be carefully prized apart with scalpels (a modern example of a medical tool having a non-medical function) and then cleaned with a brush (Bowman and Thomas 1974: 4–20).

These finds are useful because the context has been carefully recorded, and it can be asked why they were discarded in these places. It seems that there were certain areas within the fort that could be used as both a toilet and disposal for garbage. Such conditions alert us to concepts of hygiene and social rules about the disposal of waste. Indeed, when reading above, one's modern sensibility about hygiene may have been repulsed by knowing that human and animal dung were found together on the floor of a building. By modern standards, we would assume that garbage would have been disposed of outside of the fortification walls. It is possible that the structures housed animals and were regarded as an appropriate place to throw human waste and other forms of refuse. It is also possible that the area went out of use and became a zone designated for waste within the fort.

3.5.6 Stone and Bronze Inscriptions

Texts related to ancient medicine are also found on marble, stone, and bronze inscriptions (Fig. 3). Although some marble or stone inscriptions had attached to them letters that were cast in bronze, many surviving examples of these types of inscriptions are stone with lettering carved directly into the stone itself. Inscriptions are somewhat more problematic to classify, as they are, as Gordon (1983: 3) states, "at the meeting point of history and several arts". They are historical given their lettering. Yet, their shape, graphic design, and decoration are also artistic forms. The durability of the materials made them an ideal material for permanent monuments, though even these were often reused as building materials. The type of stones used for the inscriptions tended to be carved from material that was quarried locally because of weight and problems of transportation. If you are thinking that the region of origin can be determined because the stone can be provenanced, you are thinking archaeologically. Indeed, archaeologists have determined that sometimes stone was transported from regions that were further afield, where an important event might have occurred. The stone might have acted as a mnemonic device for the viewer to recall a specific incident (Bodel 2001: 20), something which is evident in how inscriptions were carved onto stones in a workshop and then placed on monuments made of different materials (Susini 1973: 23–4).

Masons carved inscriptions, though this was not always the case. Some inscriptions have been found with very rough detailing and lettering, suggesting that they were made by someone without masonry training. It was common in the manufacturing process to smooth down a flat surface, either completely or just where the text and relief sculpture were placed. Following this, horizontal lines were lightly chiselled across the flattened surface to help keep the lettering straight. The spelling is variable, and this is possibly because a draft text was given to the mason (Keppie 1991: 12–15). According to Pliny (*HN* 33.122; 40.122), cinnabar was used to make the letters more visible on walls and tombs.

Inscriptions found in situ allow us to see how they were intended to be read. For the purposes of medicine, we find altars to healing deities, doctors mentioned on grave steles, and *iamata*, which recorded the miraculous cures bestowed upon the pilgrims who visited a sanctuary – Epidauros in particular. The *iamata* were mentioned in ancient texts that described the site (e.g. Paus.

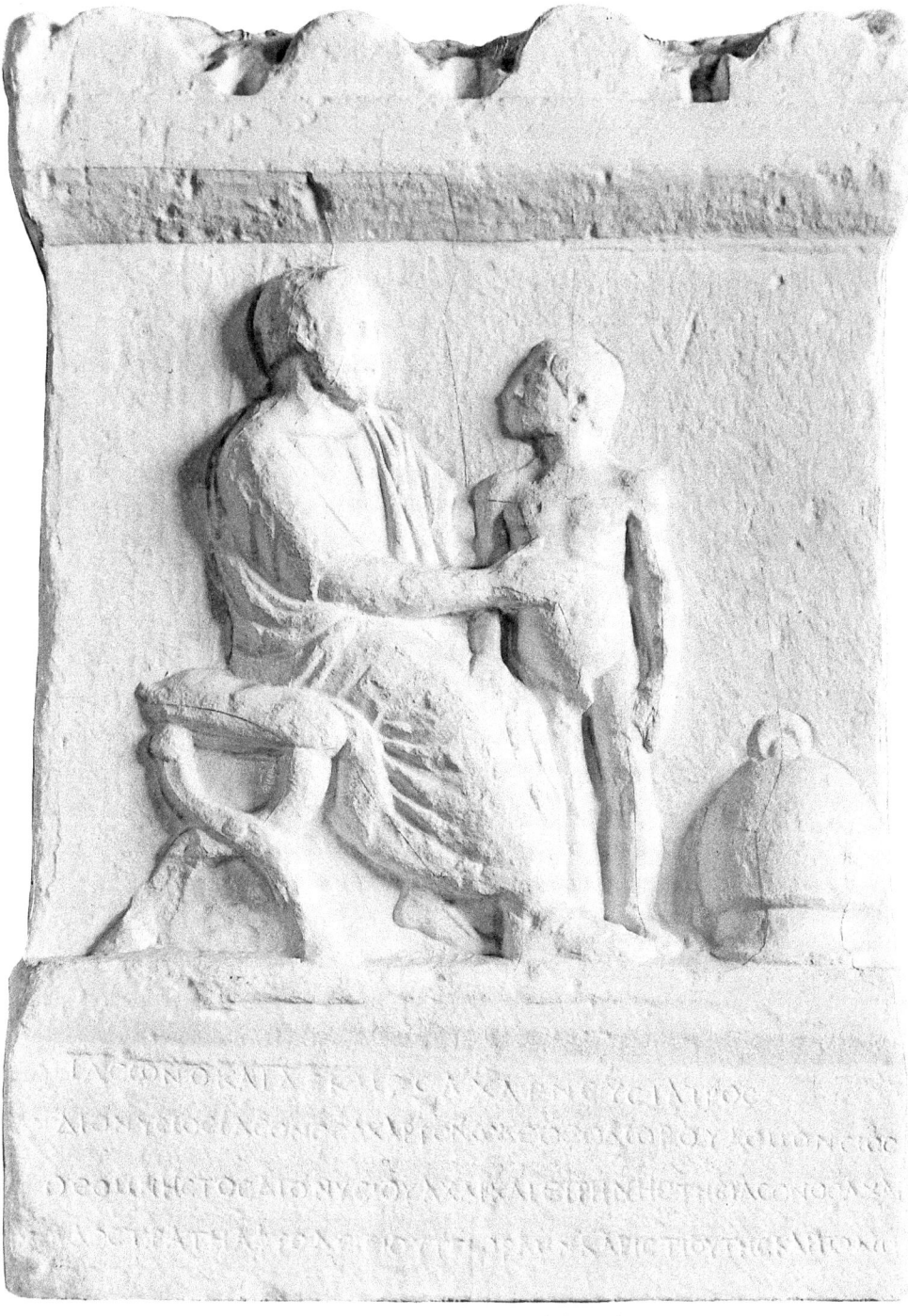

GREEK FUNERARY MONUMENT
Inscribed to Jason, also called Dehmos the Acharnian, a Physician.
It shows him palpating the liver of a patient with swollen
abdomen and wasted limbs. The ridge caused by the enlarged
liver is clearly indicated. On the right is a large cupping vessel.
II Century B.C
Original in the British Museum   R 7691
                                                  1936

3. Athenian grave stele of a Greek physician, second century AD. Courtesy of the Wellcome Library, London.

2.27.3; Str., *Geo.* 8.6.15), and they were found in the archaeological record (*IG.* IV² 1, nos. 121–2). According to Pausanias, they were displayed within the precinct of the healing sanctuary so that visitors were able to read about the problems other pilgrims suffered and the cure given to them by the deity. The central location of these implies that they were used to promote faith in the successful healing activities of the god.

Sometimes inscriptions mention the name of structures, and there is one that specifically mentions the word *valetudinarium* (hospital) from Stojnik, located in the Roman province of Moesia Superior (*CIL* III 14537=*ILS* 9147). An inscription of this sort can be of vital importance when trying to identify and determine the function of a particular building. Nonetheless, it was not found in situ, so it is impossible to link it to a particular structure. We can only say that a *valetudinarium*, whatever that was, existed, but how it was laid out, where it was located, and whether it was a single structure cannot be determined from one word on an inscription (see Baker 2002b, 2004a). On the other hand, the problem of building identification has also come to light with inscriptions dedicated to healing deities found in the courtyard of a structure at the legionary fortress at Novae. Some inscriptions to healing deities were found in a building identified as a hospital. Initially this would seem to be a useful indication of the building's function. However, found with these inscriptions were dedications to other deities who were not specifically known for their healing properties. So the question that should immediately come to mind is rather than being a hospital, could this structure or area within this structure have been a cult centre? The identification of a building based on only half of the words on inscriptions should be a warning to archaeologists to consider the whole inscription and others within the vicinity when attempting to identify the function of a structure. It also needs to be asked if the monument has been moved or reused. Finally, the date of the inscription and the date of the building need to be noted, as they might date to different periods, meaning that the function(s) of the structure could change over time.

Although not directly related to medicine, the following example further demonstrates how the location of inscription can be used to help us understand who was intended to read it. Altars to the gods Neptunus and Oceanus were found in the River Tyne in northern England, at the site of the Pons Aulius or Roman Bridge in Newcastle upon Tyne, Britain (*RIB* 1319 and 1320 respectively). The description of the two altars states that they were set up as a shrine to both gods because their location was placed at the point where the river, under the guardianship of Neptunus, met the tidal waters from the North Sea, under Oceanus. The altars were dedicated by the Legion

VI Victrix, which helped in the construction of Hadrian's Wall. Both altars were found in the north channel of the Tyne. It is possible that they eventually fell into the river, but I often wonder if they were deliberately deposited in the river by the soldiers making the dedication as a gift to the gods. It was common for votives and petitions to the god Neptune to be thrown into rivers (Tomlin 2002: 167, referencing Britanny 1997: 445, no. 1). Hence, altars might have been offered to deities in particular locations where the deity was believed to have dwelled.

3.5.7 Pottery

Ostraca, which are small pieces of broken pottery with lettering, and stamps on pottery vessels can be used to access information about medicine, in particular pharmacy. Ostraca were commonly used for tax receipts, casting votes, and by students learning to write. They were also used as tags to mark items that were transported or sold in markets (Bülow-Jacobsen 2009: 14–16). It is highly possible that medicines or medicinal ingredients might have been inscribed on ostraca, and if this were the case, it would be interesting to note the ingredients or medicines marked on them. This would not only allow one to consider the variety of materials made available throughout the Greco-Roman world but as well the distances over which the items might have been transported.

Pottery vessels sometimes had the name of the items they were intended to carry stamped or scratched onto them. An amphora with the Greek *ΠPAC* scratched on it was found at the Roman fort in Carpow, Scotland. It is believed to be short for the Greek Πρασίον (*prasion*), which translates to "horehound" (*Journal of Roman Studies* 1963: 166, no. 51), and is thought to have been wine infused with horehound. Although this interpretation is likely correct, because the full word is not given, there is no guarantee that this translation is certain. Moreover, amphorae were reused to carry other objects, such as papyri rolls, and it is plausible that something else besides the wine was delivered to the fort. If it was wine with horehound, one of its recommended uses was to cure a cough.

Another amphora found delivered to the legionary fortress of Caerleon in Wales (*Journal of Roman Studies* 1966: 224, no. 51) was marked with the letters AMINE, which is most likely short for Aminean. Aminea was a region in Apulia, Italy, that was well known in the ancient world for its fine wines. Celsus recommends the use of this wine in curing diarrhoea, and stated that wheat should be boiled in it. Subsequently, the ill person should eat the wheat on an empty stomach, followed by drinking the wine (*de Med.* 4.26.9).

Although Celsus mentions its medicinal use, it was also imbibed as a regular drink. Hence, it is much like chicken soup: it can be both a food and a medicine, and we remain uncertain as to whether the soldiers in Caerleon used it for one or both purposes. It is also plausible that the amphora had been reused, and the soldiers were left tantalized by false advertising.

In spite of the uncertainties, both amphorae were transported from places outside of Britain, and it is significant to know what the items might have meant to those who imported them. If the contents were without question, this could be used to demonstrate the possible spread of Greco-Roman pharmaceutical remedies throughout the ancient world, and determine whether some societies preferred a specific medicinal ingredient. In some cases, it is possible to take residue samples from pottery vessels to determine what was contained in them (Chapter 7), and this type of study is useful for determining if the name scratched into the vessel matches the residue.

3.5.8 Collyrium Stamps

Roman collyrium stamps were items used to mark medicines, in particular eye remedies. A number of scholars have noted the propensity of the stamps in Gaul, southern Britain, and western Germany on the border of Gaul. The information inscribed on them almost always contains three things: a person's name (possibly the doctor, owner, or maker of the medicine), the name of the medicine, and the condition(s) it was intended to cure (e.g. Baker 2011; Boon 1982; Jackson 1996; Nutton 1972; Salles 1988). The fact that they are mainly found in a certain region indicates a localized preference for either a form of medicine and/or type of object used to mark medicines. It was realized that a vast majority of them were made of green steatite and green schist, and many were recovered from areas known for votive deposition (Baker 2011). When observations were made about these aspects of the inscribed objects, new interpretations about their uses were brought to light that extended beyond the simple, functional identification of the stamp with eye medicines. They seemed to have taken on an amuletic function to protect vision. The colour green was important for the health of the eyes in the ancient world, and it is possible that those in Gaul believed that both the colour and the type of stone had healing attributes that could infuse the medicines with additional healing properties. Pliny the Elder, for example, commented upon the use of stones in healing. *Cinaedia*, a certain type of pebble, could alleviate pains in the eyes (*HN* 29.129–30), and staring at *smaragdi*, emeralds, was recommended to restore sight when the eyes were strained (Pliny, *HN* 29.132; 37.62–4).

Their place of deposition also indicated a necessary part of the healing ritual. A number of them were found in watery sources, such as rivers and wells, and it is likely that these locations were a continuation of Iron Age votive practices that occurred in Gaul. Indeed, there is ample evidence supporting the claim that there was votive deposition in water sources prior to the Roman occupation of the region (Baker 2011).

3.5.9 Lead

Pliny writes that prior to the founding of Alexandria by Alexander the Great (*HN* 13.21.69), folded pieces of lead were used for official documents. Lead is commonly known for its use in the production of curse tablets (Anderson 2002; Gager 1992). As a material, it was malleable and easy to inscribe. It was also believed to have been a cold metal, an attribute that possibly gave more power to the curse (Bodel 2001: 20). Therefore, like the green stones used for collyrium stamps, the materials upon which curses are made can play an active role in the power attributed to the inscribed words.

The provenance of lead curse tablets is widely commented upon. They are frequently found in springs, such as at the site of Bath in Britain, and in tombs where the deceased may have died violently or young, both instances in which their souls would remain restless (Gager 1992: 18–20). A papyrus fragment (*PGM* VII lines 429–58; particularly lines 432–7) of a restraining rite that could have been used to cause sickness states:

> Engrave in a plate [made] of lead from a cold-water channel what you want to happen, and when you have consecrated it with bitter aromatics such as *mrrh*, *bdellium*, styrax, and aloes and thyme, /with river mud, late in the evening or in the middle of the night, where there is a stream or the drain of a bath, having tied a cord [to the plate] throw it into the stream or into the sea – [and let it be] carried along.

The excerpt from this papyrus fragment supports what has been found in the archaeological record, and explains that the quality of the material was important. It also informs the reader that certain activities had to be carried out at specific times. Hence, the manufacture of the object and the manner in which it was to be treated were necessary for the efficacy of the spell.

3.5.10 Writing Materials

Since it is possible that the materials on which something was written might have had healing powers or the ability to cause illness, one also needs to question what types of materials were used for writing and whether they could have had properties that might have imbued the work with some form of healing potential.

Inks used on papyrus, wood tablets, and parchment were commonly made of soot that was mixed with gum arabic. From the third/second BC onwards, mordent metallic inks were also used in writing. These inks were made from powdered gall nuts, a metallic salt of iron or copper, along with gum arabic, and water. The Indian inks made from soot black and gum arabic did not fade, unlike those made of iron-gall, which turned from black to brown over time. The inks were generally processed into blocks or in inkwells. When formed into blocks, the ink was suspended in water, and a brush was used for the document. The ink also could have been supplied in an ink bottle, while a quill or reed with a pointed end would have been used as the writing implement (Bülow-Jacobsen 2009: 18). It is possible to make a chemical analysis of the inks to see if certain ones were used for different types of texts, although I am unaware of any study of this kind in relation to medical texts. But given the possibility of doing so, it can be asked what significance the ingredients of the ink had, and why it was necessary to use them on specific objects, much like the use of certain stones or lead, as mentioned above.

3.6 TEXT AS MATERIAL CULTURE

To draw together our considerations above, and at the risk of repetition, it is worthwhile emphasizing that when conducting any form of investigation of the past, texts should be considered as material culture. Besides the materials on which the texts were written, the act of writing and the words themselves may have held significances that extend beyond the defined meaning of the words. There exist some interesting discussions on the "non-utilitarian", or what Bodel (2001: 19) refers to as the "symbolic", connotations of words on various types of documents. This issue is discussed here mainly to draw the reader's attention to the fact that texts are not always directly translatable or that words can take on other functions besides conveying their linguistic denotations. When considering documents from an archaeological perspective, it is vital to compare their material properties with the text written on them. And deliberation also needs to be given to the fact that words are a form of material culture in themselves that assume meanings/functions in relation to their cultural and situational context.

Beard has convincingly argued that the Arval Brethren, a college of priests dedicated to worshipping the fertility goddess Dea Dia just outside of Rome, would annually inscribe their ritual to the goddess at the site where they worshipped. Although the recorded information became more detailed over time, the same course of events was always explained. When no space remained on the tablets for further inscription, the furniture within the sanctuary was then used to record the event. Since it was repetitive, the act of inscribing does not appear to have been carried out for someone to read or to provide instructions for new priests, but rather it appears to have been a necessary part of the ritual itself (Beard 1985: 139–41).

Another act where the written words have other non-denotational meanings occurs in *damnatio memoriae*. This was the removal of a person's name from a monument if they had fallen out of favour. The name was usually scratched or carved out of the stone or metal, and the faces were removed from sculptures and paintings. The deletions left visible scars that would most likely have caused the condemned to be remembered in a poor light rather than being forgotten (Bodel 2001: 23).

It also seems that uttering the name of a deity or a foreign word or phrase might have been thought to carry certain weight, and perhaps acted as part of a medical cure. Lucian of Samosata (*Philops.* 9–10) wrote about a debate between Tychiades and Deinomachus, where Tychiades says that he does not believe that the use of a god's name or foreign phrase can cause a fever or inflammation to flee from the body in spite of the fact that he believes in the gods. This story suggests that there were those in the ancient world who believed a foreign word could be uttered as part of an incantation. This idea is not limited to the text in question. As Versnel (2002) has demonstrated, these ideas are found in other forms of Roman literature that discuss cures for illnesses and accidents (see also Frankfurter 1994). In addition to this, Faraone (2009) shows that Iambic metre was employed in the use of protective charms and chants. Therefore, the act of writing, the use of words themselves, and the metre in which they were chanted could be a socially manipulated "object".

3.7 CONCLUSION

In conclusion, I would like to end this chapter with an example of a phylactery that is described on a Greek magical papyrus for the preservation of health (*PGM* VII. 579–90). It neatly summarizes the various aspects of text as a form of material culture mentioned in this chapter.

> A phylactery, a bodyguard against daimons, against phantasms, /against every sickness and suffering, to be written on a leaf of gold or silver or tin or on hieratic papyrus. When worn it works mightily for it is the name

of power of the great god and his seal, and it is as follows "KMĒPHIS CHPHYRIS IAEŌ IAŌ AEĒ IAŌ OŌ AIŌN IAEŌBAPHRENE/ MOUNOTHILARIKRIPHIAE Y EAIPHIRKIRALITHANYOMENERP HABŌEAI. These are the names; the figure is like this: let the Snake be biting its tail, the names being written inside [the circle made by] the snake, and the characters, thus as follows (drawing of figures)

The whole figure is [drawn] thus, as given below, with [the spell] "Protect my Body, [and] the/entire soul of me, NN". And when you have consecrated [it], wear [it].

The information on this papyrus tells us a lot about the manner of inscription and use of words. First, we are told how to make an object that will be worn to protect someone's health. Then we learn that it has to be written on specific materials. It is therefore possible that the materials are not only durable, but may hold some importance in themselves in order for the charm to work. Magical words and symbols must be written on it. These are foreign words or "nonsense" words that cannot be translated, but hold a meaning important for the efficacy of the ritual. The object has to be consecrated, presumably by chanting the spell, though other actions may have been required. Thus, we can see that the words, the materials, and the place where the words were to be sworn explain that the written object has a meaning and function that would not be discernible if the phylactery was found without the instructions and was only translated.

The materials discussed all have textual elements that pertain to healing, disease, and treatments in the ancient world. By expanding examinations to consider their archaeological properties, their social meaning can become apparent. On one level, it is possible to learn about trade and the jobs involved in producing materials and in writing documents. On another level, we can see what texts were deemed important enough to copy, how they were meant to be read, and how the materials might have helped in their ability to cause or cure illness. These concerns provide us with insights into Greco-Roman perceptions of medical scholarship and practices that cannot be accessed through the texts alone.

Box 2. Accessing Collections of Textual Remains

Anyone wishing to study papyri fragments and inscriptions can consult the vast corpora dedicated to the publication of these remains, some of which are mentioned in the further reading section of this chapter. For example, Latin inscriptions are found in the Corpus of Latin inscriptions *CIL*, Greek in the *IG* and *CIG*. Coins are published in numismatic collections. Medical inscriptions and papyri fragments have also been gathered together in specific collections. In the 1930s, Gummerus published the inscriptions mentioning doctors known at the time. Although more inscriptions have come to light since the publication, it is still a useful source for beginning any examination of medical inscriptions. Some more recent works of medical inscriptions are Rémy (1984, 1991) and Rémy and Faure (2010), who list those found in the north-western provinces, and Flemming (2000: 383–91), who lists *medica* or female medics. Some of the most well-known inscriptions for healing are the *iamata*, particularly those found at Epidauros (Edelstein and Edelstein 1988 [1945]). Between 200 and 300 Greek papyri with medical contents are currently known, and there is a project underway collecting and republishing medical papyri in the *Corpus dei Papyri Greci di Medicina* (Andorlini 1997, 2001–; Jones 2009: 354). Other items, such as collyrium stamps have been catalogued in Voinot's collection of 1999.

Some of the collections are more detailed than others. If a thorough account of the textual source is provided, one would expect to find an entry to contain information about the object's archaeological provenance, the condition of the material, a discussion of the handwriting style in which it was written, a date, and sometimes an image or description of decoration if there were any found with the text. Sometimes the archaeological provenance is given, but for the most part we are only told an object was found at a certain site rather than details of the exact location or whether it was recovered with other objects. When this information is not provided in the catalogue, it may still be possible to access it. In these instances, if it is known where the inscription, papyrus, or coin was originally excavated, it may be mentioned or described in the original site report. Sometimes reports are published but leave out vital information. If this should be the case or if the information was never published (also a sad reality of certain archaeological sites), it might still be possible to obtain the information required if it is known where the original site reports and collections are archived – usually in a museum, university, or perhaps a special collection of a university library. A request can be made to consult the materials first-hand. It should be remembered that some archaeologists are more thorough with their record keeping than others. A general rule of thumb is that the earlier a site was excavated, the less likely it is that a record of an artefact's location or associated artefacts was kept.

CONSIDERATION QUESTIONS

1. Visit your library and find an inscription, papyrus fragment, letter, or other form of inscribed remain that is relevant to ancient medicine. Consider all of its aspects: archaeological and textual. Ask whether there might have been a correlation between the textual details and the archaeological properties of the surviving excerpt.

2. Consider whether academics can competently use two sources of evidence in their research – that is, material remains and texts. How might they overcome some problems of methodology?

FURTHER READING

Bagnall, R., ed. 2009. *The Oxford Handbook of Papyrology.* Oxford: Oxford University Press.

Deetz, J. 1996 (rev. ed.). *In Small Things Forgotten.* New York: Anchor Press/Doubleday.

Edelstein, E. J., and L. Edelstein 1988 [1945]. *Asclepius: Collection and Interpretation of the Testimonies.* Baltimore, MD: Johns Hopkins University Press.

Keppie, L. 1991. *Understanding Roman Inscriptions.* London: B. T. Batsford.

Inscriptions

AE   *L'Année Épigraphique: Revue des Publications Épigraphiques Relatives à l'antiqué Romaine.* Paris 1888– .

CIG   *Corpus Inscriptionum Graecarum.* Berlin: Könliglich Preussische Akademie der Wissenschaften zu Berlin.

CIL   *Corpus Inscriptionum Latinorum.* Consilio et Ductoritate Academie Litterarum Regiae Borussial Edition. Berlin: Academieder Wissenschaften1862–.

Gummerus, H. 1932. *Der Ärztesstand im römischen Reiche nach dem Inschriften.* Helsinki: Akademische Buchhandlung.

IG   *Inscriptiones Graecae.* Berlin: Brandenburgische Akademie der Wissenschaften.

IGRR   *Inscriptiones Graecae ad Res Romanas Pertinentes: Auctoritate et Impensis Academiae Inscriptionum et litterarum humaniarum.* R. L. V. Cagnet and J. F. Toutain (eds.) Rome: L'Erma Bretschneider 1964.

ILS   *Inscriptiones Latinae Selectae,* H. Dessau, ed. 1892–1916. Berlin: Apud Weidmannos.

Rémy, B. 1984. "Les Inscriptions de médecins en Gaule", *Gallia* 42: 115–52.

    1991. "Les Inscriptions de médicines dans les provinces romaines de la péninsule ibérique", *REA* 93: 321–64.

Rémy, B., and P. Faure 2010. *"Les Médecines dans l'Occident romain: Péninsule Ibérique, Bretagne, Gaules, Germaines".* Paris: Ausonius Publications: Scripta Antiqua 27, Ausonius, Pessac/Diffusion de Boccard.

RIB   *The Roman Inscriptions of Britain,* R. G. Collingwood and R. P. Wright, eds. Stroud: Alan Sutton 1995.

Papyri Collections

http://library.duke.edu/rubenstein/scriptorium/papyrus/texts/clist_ostraca.html (this is an invaluable list of reference materials)

http://www.papyri.info/

PGM   Betz, H. D. 1996. *Greek Magical Papyri in Translation.* Chicago: University of Chicago Press.

P.Mich   Papyri in the University of Michigan Collection. Ann Arbor: University of
              Michigan Press
P.Oxy   B. Grenfell, A. S. Hunter, et al., eds. *The Oxyrhynchus Papyri*. London 1898–.
P. Rainer   *Papyrus Erzherzog Rainer der Papyrussammlung der Österreichischen Nationalbibliothek.*
              Vienna: Verlag Brüder Hollinek 1883–.

Vindolanda Tablets

Bowman, A. K., and J. D. Thomas 1994. *The Vindolanda Writing Tablets (Tabulae Vindolandenses II).*
    London: British Museum Press.
Bowman, A. K., J. D. Thomas, and R. S. O. Tomlin 2011. "The Vindolanda Writing-Tablets
    (Tabulae Vindolandenses IV, Part 2)", *Britannia* 42: 113–44.

CHAPTER 4

IMAGES

4.1 INTRODUCTION

In the previous chapter, it was shown that textual remains could be examined as material culture. It was thought best to introduce the examination of archaeological remains with the types of materials a medical historian would recognize. Yet, texts are probably not what most people would think of when asked to describe archaeological remains. So now we turn to materials that are more commonly found in books on archaeology to show how they can be studied for their medical attributes.

In this chapter, I employ a "proper" archaeological method to the study of images. The reason for this is because art history and the study of images, rather than small-scale objects, is the foundation upon which classical archaeology is based. Moreover, the dating system used in this subfield of archaeology is constituted by the evolution of artistic styles and techniques seen in Greek and Roman art. It is essential for anyone interested in the archaeology of the Greco-Roman world to have a basic background in the traditional methods of study because a majority of the materials described in published works are classified as forms of art, such as sculptures, architectural details, and vase paintings. These objects can be examined in terms of style and narrative, but they can also be used to ascertain information about medical practices, understandings of a healthy body, and images of doctors and healing deities, for example.

This chapter begins with a discussion of the history of classical archaeology to familiarize the reader with the developments that have occurred in the subject. Along with this, some recent approaches to the anthropology of art will be presented because they have forced us to realize that cultural aesthetics differ between societies, and our modern classifications of art might not have been the same as that of the Greeks and Romans. Acknowledging this allows for new ways of defining and examining art objects, helping classical archaeology to move beyond a traditional art historical approach. This last feature of innovation is important, since it allows the archaeologist to envision medical history in ways that are less local to his or her own time period. Once the history and theories are explained, the third part of the chapter will explore how images related to medicine can be examined in the light of more recent theoretical considerations of art objects.

Before turning to the role of art history, a few precursory comments should be made with respect to the manner in which the archaeology of the Greco-Roman period is art historical. To see this, one need only consider how university classes concerned with this period are offered in classics, art history, and archaeology departments under such titles as "Greek Art and Architecture" and "Roman Art and Architecture". Core textbooks associated with these courses focus on architecture, sculptures, mosaics, frescos, vase paintings, statuettes, and "minor arts", such as numismatics and jewellery (e.g. Boardman 1996; Henig 1995; Pedley 1998; Ramage and Ramage 2000). The material is often presented chronologically with attention given to style and narrative. Students emerge from these classes well versed in the ability to identify and date significant monuments and works of art, name the artist or architect of a particular sculpture or building, and recognize artistic techniques and styles. They are also able to place each work in its sociohistorical context and identify the mythological and/or historical narratives of the images. Since classical archaeology is grounded in art history, little attention has been given to the archaeological remains that tell us about the daily activities of people living at the time, which is quite unlike the archaeology of other periods (see Snodgrass 2007: 15–17 and Whitley 2001 for fuller details). Although the methodology of the subject is evolving to incorporate other forms of archaeological remains and interpretative approaches, these have been slow to catch on.

While the art historical approach dominates classical archaeology, it is not the aim of this chapter to provide descriptions of artistic styles from the period. This information is readily available in introductory books on the art and architecture of Greece and Rome. Additionally, if this were a critical book on Greco-Roman art, full consideration of a definition of art in the Greco-Roman world would be required. This question is extremely interesting, but answering it is tangential to the purpose of this chapter. Instead, being aware of the fact that there were divergent definitions of art is sufficient in helping us to escape the confines of stylistic approaches to the remains. If the cliché "a picture is worth a thousand words" is true, then the aim of this chapter can be seen as "reading" the art containing medical and pharmaceutical illustrations as a way of better understanding medical history. Thus, explanations of how these images can be studied will be given to see what the "thousand words" can tell us about medical practices in the past.

4.2 ART HISTORY AND CLASSICAL ARCHAEOLOGY

Although Greco-Roman images are classified under modern Western definitions of high art, this distinction does not correspond to Greek definitions of art. In the ancient world, art was defined as a *techne* (skill or craft), just like medicine. The muses inspired poetry, music, and dance; they did not help in the creation of images. These fell under the remit of the goddess Athena and the god Hephaistos whose crafts were basically what we would refer to today as applied arts (Boardman 1996: 14–16). In spite of this, we still categorize ancient images as forms of high art, and this stems from the history of the subject's development.

The methods used in studying classical archaeology can be traced to the publication of Johann Joachim Winckelmann's work *Geschichte der Kunst des Alterthums* (*History of Art of Antiquity*) in 1764. When attempting to make sense of the thousands of statues and images that had survived from antiquity, Winckelmann established a classificatory system that was based on schemes used for dating literature. The dating system was divided into four main periods: the archaic period, which roughly dates to the sixth century BC; the high classical period, dating to the fifth and fourth centuries BC; the Hellenistic, or beautiful era, dating from the death of Alexander the Great to the Roman era; and the Roman era, which was referred to as the style of imitators. Prior to the establishment of this dating system, the material from the Greco-Roman period was simply referred to as "antique". To Winckelmann, Greek art from the high classical period was the zenith upon which art from other places and periods was to be measured, believing its decline began after the death of Alexander the Great (Beard and Henderson 2001: 68–71; Ramage and Ramage 2000: 22; Snodgrass 2007: 17; Whitley 2001: 20–3).

Over time, some alterations were made to his system of dating, but it remains the framework upon which archaeological finds from the period are classified. The periods are now divided as follows: archaic (600–500 BC); classical, which is divided into early, middle, and late (c. 500/490–322 BC); and Hellenistic (322–31 BC). Roman art is categorized by the Republican (c. 200–31/27 BC), Imperial (31/27 BC to Diocletian in AD 284), and late Roman/Late Antique periods (the fifth or sixth centuries; see Tables 1 and 2). The dating is now seen as more or less provisional, with revisions and moderations open to argumentation.

TABLE 1. *Greek Art Dates*

Period Name	Dates	Style
Archaic	600–500/480 BC	Movement and balance develop in the human form
Early Classical	500/480–450 BC	The human form becomes more realistic and bodily movements are depicted
High Classical	450–430 BC	The idealized human form.
Late Classical	430–323 BC	More fluid styles and movement
Early Hellenistic	323–275 BC	Royal iconography
Middle Hellenistic	275–150 BC	Hellenistic baroque, influences from Egypt and the eastern kingdoms
Late Hellenistic	150–31 BC	Diversity, neo-classicism

TABLE 2. *Roman Art Dates*

Period Name	Date	Styles
Republican	200–31/27 BC	Verism; Hellenistic influences
Imperial Roman (divided into periods based on imperial dynasties and emperors)	31/27 BC–Time of Dicoletian	
Augustan	31 BC–AD 14	Classical Greek and Hellenistic influences
Julio-Claudian	AD 14–68	Classical Greek influences; under Claudius (AD 41–54), there was a return to Italian or rustic styles
Flavians	AD 69–98	Verism and military triumphs
Trajan	AD 98–117	Military triumphs
Hadrian	AD 117–138	Classical Greek revival
Antonines	AD 138–193	Changes to regional styles
Severans	AD 193–235	African influences
The Soldier Emperors	AD 235–284	Military portraits
Tetrarchs	AD 284–312	A move away from individualism
Late Antique/Late Roman	AD 312–	Early Christian forms

Contributing to the establishment of a chronological sequence was the identification of the artist. For the purpose of archaeological identification, sometimes a date and work by a particular artist were used as a point of reference. Then, for example, other sculptures similar in style could be attributed to that artist and/or period. One of the main proponents of this type of classification was Adolf Furtwängler, who lived in the nineteenth century (Snodgrass 2007: 19–20). Developing from this method was the creation of large-scale catalogues of art objects, such as the kind undertaken by Beazley in his study of Greek vase painting (Snodgrass 2007: 21–3). Like Furtwängler, Beazley was concerned with examining the technical style to determine both the artist who created the image on the vessel and its date.

Although potters were considered to be on the lower echelons of Greek society (pots and pottery sherds survive in vast quantities), the vessels are referred to as vases and their paintings were given and still hold the status of high art.

In 1994, the classification of pottery vessels as vases was challenged by Vickers and Gill who contended that the objects were not forms of high art because they were likely copies of metal vessels made for less cost and were therefore more common. This is not to say that the images are unworthy of examination; on the contrary, they are a valuable resource for gaining insights into Greek daily life. The scenes, for example, often depict activities that are rarely, if ever, mentioned in literature.

In spite of these and other challenges, the approaches to classifying Greek art remain influenced by the early attempts described above. This has largely to do with the way in which Greek art was conceived to be original in its technique and content. Approaches to Roman art, on the other hand, have developed differently.

4.2.1 Roman Art

Unlike Greek art, Roman art was seen by Winckelmann as a period of imitators because many copies of Greek sculptures were made in the Roman period. For example, some Roman statues, such as the Augusts of Prima Porta, are based on Greek sculptural techniques. While Winckelmann's judgement subsequently led to Roman art being considered by some scholars as less important than Greek art, this inferior designation naturally opened broader questions about Roman art and its influences. If art from the Roman period was simply derivative, could it be called "Roman" art? Did it have one source or many? Some of the arguments put forth about the definition of Roman art are described in Otto Brendel's *Prolegomena to the Study of Roman Art* (1979; see also Elsner's discussion in Hölscher 2004: xv–xxxi). Some suggestions found in Brendel are that Roman art is eclectic because it includes styles from around the Roman Empire and from different periods, and early Christian because some stylistic elements found in Christian art were developed in the imperial period. In many respects, Roman art encompasses a number of elements and was, like other periods, clearly influenced by the social and political events of the time in which it was produced (e.g. Elsner 1995, 1996; Ramage and Ramage 2000; Zanker 1990).

In contrast to the designation of Greek art as a form of "high art", the "lower status" afforded to Roman art has, in some respects, freed academics of Roman studies from the confines of traditional approaches to classical archaeology. Hence, the field of Roman art, and ultimately archaeology in terms of small finds and structures, has been more open to interpretations using new theoretical methodologies. Having said this, however, there is still a strong tradition of studying the art objects, as frescos, mosaics, sculptures, and monumental structures have tended to receive a considerable amount of scholarly attention.

Another factor that has contributed to developments in Roman scholarship involves historical circumstance. According to Millett, classical archaeology, particularly Roman archaeology, developed differently in Europe in comparison to the United States. Originally, classics was studied in elite schools in both the United States and Europe. However, following the Second World War, European countries were dealing with large-scale economic instability and obstacles to rebuilding their social infrastructure. This led to the breakdown of some traditional social-class barriers, or what Millett (2007: 39) refers to as a "democratization" process in scholarship. Democratization had another effect besides providing students in state schools with an opportunity to learn classics. There was, as well, a broadening of theoretical approaches in which disciplinary boundaries were more permeable. For example, open dialogue between Romanists and prehistorians enabled Romanists to widen their theoretical methods and consider a broader range of materials. It also led to the development of a thriving field of provincial Roman archaeology in Europe, which has ties to scholarship on pre- and protohistory. This is evident with the development of the *Theoretical Roman Archaeology Conference* (TRAC) in 1991 (Scott 1993).

In America, however, the expansion of theoretical outlooks did not occur. Without the same wartime devastation, the elite approach to classics persisted, and classical archaeology remained distinct from anthropology and contract archaeology. As well, study of the Roman provinces was often omitted due to the perception that provinces were not a part of Rome "proper". With the lack of new theoretical outlooks from other fields of archaeology, Greek and Roman archaeology in America are still studied from a classical art historical approach (Millett 2007: 38–9). Nonetheless, it is impossible to remain in a theoretical bubble for very long, and as we will consider below, some changes within the field have occurred over the last century.

4.2.2 Art Historical Developments

Developments in archaeological interpretations, although slower to evolve in classical archaeology, have still had some impact on the manner in which the subject is studied. In this section, we will look at examples from processualist and postprocessualist archaeology, iconology, and a hermeneutic approach sensitive to use of anachronistic concepts.

Processualist archaeology has influenced studies about the technology and tools used in creating sculptures and paintings (Boardman 1996: 26). For example, archaeologists were not originally concerned with the process of producing artefacts, but more in the finished objects themselves. Processualists look specifically at the methods involved in creating the artefacts from a scientific viewpoint – such as the types of drilling techniques used to make the curls of hair in a sculpture. Critically reacting to this approach, postprocessualism moved away from questions of methods of production and towards what it viewed to be more significant to the creation process – in this case, gender and sexuality and how they were depicted in art (Clarke 1998; Stewart 1997).

The method of classification used by Wincklemann is often referred to as the iconographical approach or, as discussed above, the description of the styles, forms, dating, and mythological or historical narratives relating to the art object. Critical revision of this method came in the form of the iconological approach, which is interested in the historical and social context in which the work was made (Elsner in Hölscher 2004: xxii). For example, the sculpture of the Augustan age (31 BC–AD 14) has been studied for its role in political propaganda, one interpretation being that the sculpture presented the idea that an empire, rather than republic, was beneficial for the people of Rome (Zanker 1990). Another example is seen in the effect that the Persian War had on the style of mid-fifth-century Athenian architectural design. The Athenian Parthenon is a perfect instance of Athenian pride in their victory over the Persians. It was built on a grand scale, and its relief sculpture incorporated scenes of citizens parading, possibly for the Panathenaic festival. The placement of human beings on a monument dedicated to Athena would never have been done in different political circumstances because here we see mortals in the position of deities (Pollitt 1972: 68–95).

Numerous images from the period survive, and they can be a useful source of evidence to access different aspects of life in the ancient world. Conventionally, however, the interpretations made of these surviving works tend to suppose that people living in the Greco-Roman world would have had a definition of art and aesthetics similar to our own. This has not only led to the use of anachronistic standards, but it also assumes the meanings of the images are transparent or easily accessible despite the historical distance of the Greeks and the Romans. Some recent scholarship has demonstrated that, even in the Roman period, understandings of the images would have differed depending on social contexts, and in light of this, we should be forewarned not to make interpretations with our own standards and aesthetical points of view. Elsner, for instance, uses an example of a fish to show various readings of an image in a close period of time. He says that an early Christian might see the fish as having a symbolic meaning associated with Christ, while a pagan would see it as a source of food or something found in the natural world (Elsner 1995: 3). Other studies have shown regional differences in artistic representation, indicating the existence of various perceptions of imagery across the Greco-Roman world (see, e.g., Henig 2000, and papers in Scott and Webster 2003). As the field of study is becoming more open to different approaches to critical analysis, new questions are being asked about the materials that extend beyond date, narrative, and style.

In spite of more recent challenges and discussions to the subject, the traditional methods still influence the foundation upon which the subject is taught and, in many cases, has continued to be researched (e.g. Shanks 1995; Snodgrass 2007). However, if we want to learn more about what art objects meant to the people of the time in which they were created and what they might tell us about life in the past, we should be asking how these images can be looked at beyond style and narrative. Is there a scholarly precedent for considering such an approach?

4.3 ANTHROPOLOGY OF ART

While in the modern West, sculptures, paintings, and other decorative features are classified as art and are viewed for their styles and narrative, anthropological studies of art have taught us that these definitions and readings do not always apply to decorated objects and images made and viewed by societies outside of the West. Through anthropology, it has also been demonstrated that art objects can change their meanings over time. For instance, Oosten (1992) informs us that when examining Inuit masks from the nineteenth century, we cannot ask modern Inuits about the meanings the masks held for their ancestors. Although it is possible that some ideas about them were maintained over a long period of time, changes in beliefs, newly introduced ideas, and even events, for example, can all influence how people think and understand objects and images. This warns us that the Greeks and Romans would have also understood their art objects in a different manner than we do. Given the geographical scale of the Greco-Roman world, object meanings might also have varied between places.

By not introducing our own concepts of art when understanding foreign objects, anthropologists have realized images might be classed as something other than art and can hold diverse meanings and functions to those
who make, use, and view them. Because of this recognition, anthropologists
approach the study of art objects from multivariant points of view. This has
also made them keenly aware of the fact that they must try and divorce themselves from their own cultural biases and categories when studying decorated
objects from other societies.

In the light of this observation, Gell (1994: 42) argued that in order for
art objects to be studied in a different society, a break from Western aesthetics must be made. Gell suggested that we should consider the agency
of the artist and the skills they employed in creating the piece in order to
ascertain how and why it was made. Such considerations also inform us as to
whether the actual task of creating the object played a significant role in the
object's function. For example, Gell noticed that objects are sometimes made
to serve purposes beyond simple decoration or narrative. In his examination of Trobriand canoe-boards, the act of creating the decoration helped to
empower the object with properties that would make the decorations "dazzle"
those with whom they traded. This "magical art" allowed the Trobriands to
obtain more goods when they were trading than they might otherwise have
done (Gell 1994: 44). In comparison to ancient medicine, images drawn on
medical objects and Greek magical papyri might have served a similar purpose, like the words discussed in the previous chapter. Both the act of drawing the image and the image itself could have affected the magic of the papyri
and helped with healing.

As with the question of defining Greek and Roman art mentioned above,
the anthropology of art is an interesting area of study, and is beginning to
have a wider impact on ancient art. Indeed, the point can never be under-
stated that art objects can take on various meanings and functions that do not
correspond with our understandings and classifications. To break from this,
the following section will be used to explain how archaeologists can address
the meanings and roles of images. To begin, some traditional methods of
assessment will be presented in order to familiarize the reader with how the
scholarship on images is conventionally undertaken. In contrast, anthropological approaches will be discussed in order to understand the importance of
social attitudes towards certain aspects of medicine and the role of the image
in medical treatments. Another benefit of these approaches is how they can
be compared to literary sources to see if the images and the literature support
one another, or if different views become apparent.

4.4 GENERAL QUESTIONS TO BE ADDRESSED
OF ART OBJECTS

When setting out to examine images, there are a few general aspects about them that need to be recorded by the archaeologist. (1) The image must be classified according to its type: a statue in the round, a relief sculpture, or fresco painting, for example. (2) Once classified, descriptions of the image should be documented. The archaeologist should note who or what is being depicted and any other objects or scenery included with it. (3) If possible, it is important to try to identify the artist. (4) The date and provenance of the work should be recorded.

In relation to the first point, it is generally easy to identify the type of object. However, the remaining three points require some explanation. Many images from the Greco-Roman period depict deities, leaders, prominent individuals, and scenes from daily life. Sometimes names are painted on or inscribed in the images, making it easy to identify who was being portrayed. Yet, there are many instances where no names were given. In this case, the image may be recognized by its attributes. Certain deities have an animal, particular item of clothing, or an event with which they are associated. Asclepius, for example, was commonly depicted bearded, holding a staff, usually with a snake wrapped around it (Fig. 4). Sometimes names are applied to an image simply because it was found in a site associated with a particular deity. In other instances, identifications are made because they look similar to those that were more positively identified. However, this latter means of identifying images is extremely problematic. To test this, one needs only to look through catalogues of images without reading the identification given to the deity. One may be disconcerted as to how common it is to confuse deities. Images said to be Somnus and Hypnos found in the *LIMC* (*Lexicon Iconographicum Mythologiae Classicae*) have similar attributes to Asclepius and Hygieia.

In regards to the third point, in some instances it is possible to identify the artist who created the image and/or the person who commissioned it. This information is occasionally found on dedicatory inscriptions. This will also help the archaeologist consider, along with its date and style, what political, social, and philosophical circumstances might have influenced the design and form of the work.

As noted with the fourth point, the archaeologist should also record the date and provenance of the image. Dating is important not only for identifying certain stylistic designs, but it also acts as a guide to make comparisons between different periods. For example, a scholar may wish to know if snakes were more commonly associated with the god Asclepius at particular times or in places. In this way, it is also possible to consider whether certain narratives were more popular in specific places and times. There might also be indications that understandings of healing deities were regionally and temporally specific. Identifying the provenance of an art object allows archaeologists to determine how it was intended to be viewed. A secure provenance can help identify whether it was meant for public or private viewing.

4.5 SPECIFIC QUESTIONS TO BE ADDRESSED

Once an archaeologist has recorded the general information described above, it is possible for them to ask more particular questions about the objects. In this section, we will explore the pertinent questions that can be raised in order to learn about ancient medical practices.

4.5.1 How Was the Image Intended to be Viewed?

As mentioned above, the provenance of an object can help us to determine how an image might have been viewed in the ancient world. Many of the images archaeologists study were found in public contexts, largely because public buildings and sites were locations that called for adornment. Since there was very likely a higher rate of illiteracy than today, the placement of images in different contexts could also act as "advertisements" for the work carried out in an area. Images can also act as a reminder of a specific event, or help in identifying a particular place or group of people. Images of healing deities on altars and monuments can indicate who was being worshipped in particular areas, and give us an idea of how the gods and their actions were understood. Asclepius was known for treating people while they slept, and an image of him healing someone sleeping was found at the Asclepion in Piraeus (Fig. 5). It dates to the fourth century BC, and the god is identifiable because he is larger in scale than the others, and is standing over a sleeping patient.

The scene can also be examined to see how healing spaces might have appeared. Figure 5, for example, shows a couch or *kline*, and while this gives us an idea of how a sanctuary might have been furnished, one should also bear in mind that one image cannot be used as a universal representation of how *all* sanctuaries were furnished. With a view towards archaeological identification, images that show scenes of sanctuaries can be used to reconstruct fragmentary remains of small finds. For example, when parts of

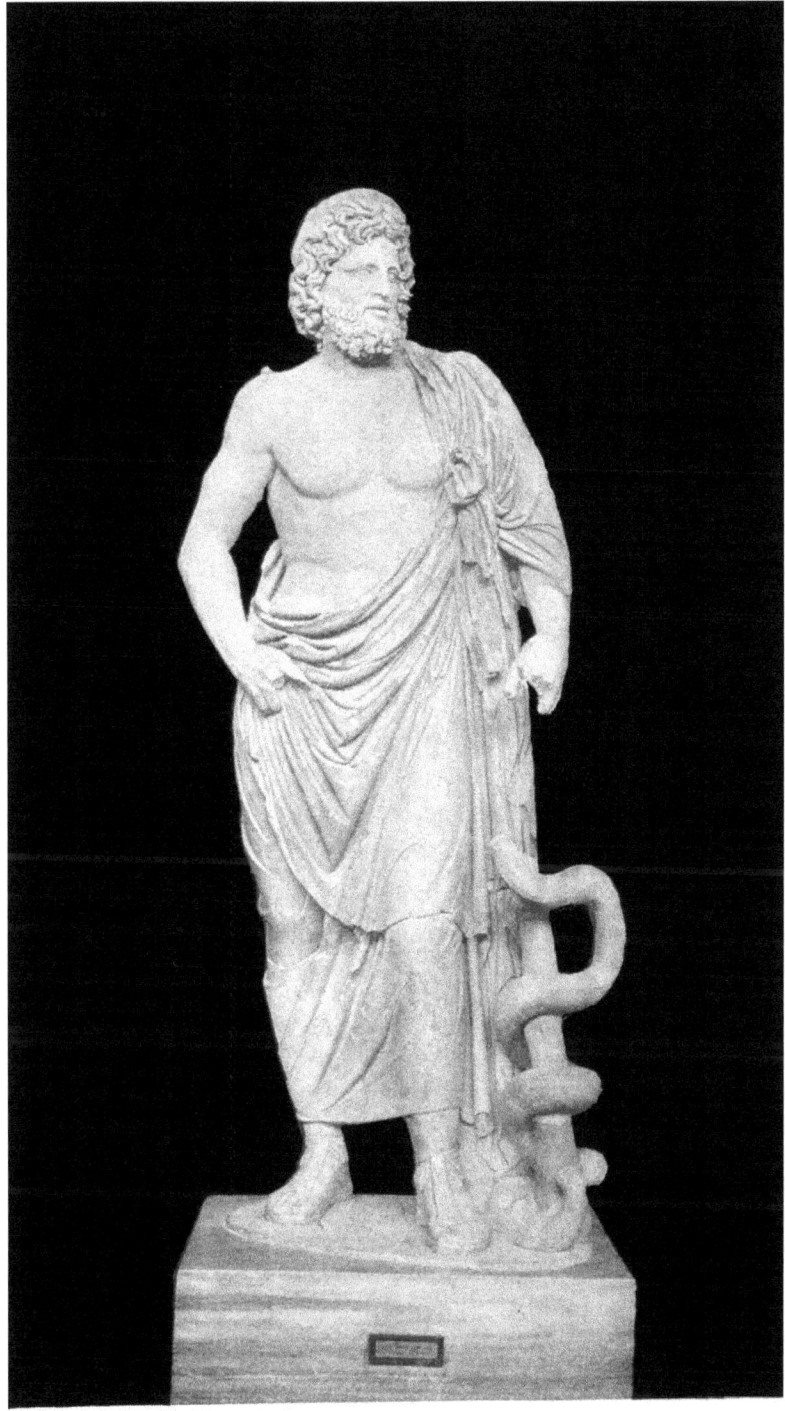

ASKLEPIOS
The antient Greek deity of healing

4. Statue of Asclepius from Epidauros. Courtesy of the Wellcome Library, London.

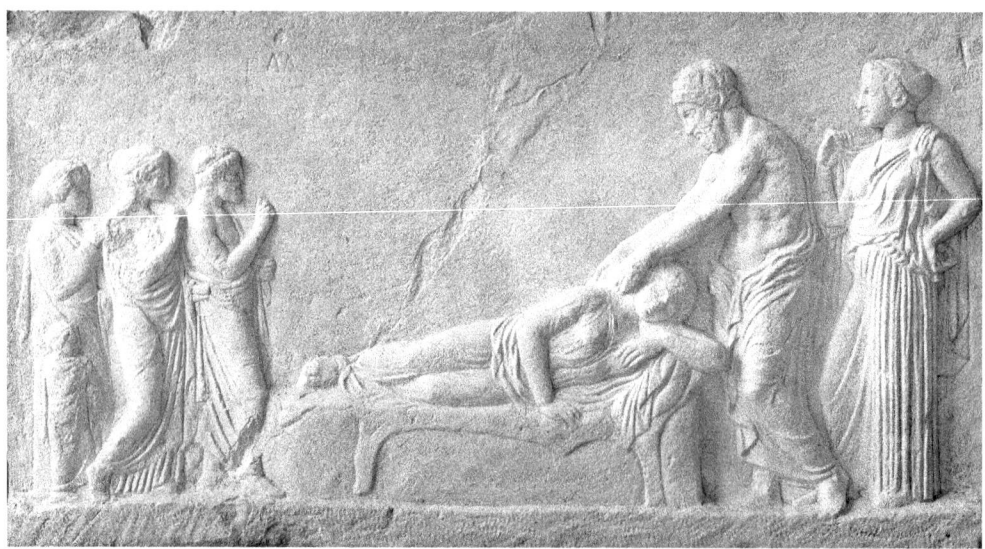

5. Fragment of a relief from the Asclepion at Piraeus, fourth century BC. Courtesy of the Wellcome Library, London.

furniture are found in the archaeological record, they can be compared to these representations to give us an idea of how they may have looked when complete.

Pictures on coins were another means by which messages can be conveyed about a person or place, since they were widely distributed in the ancient world. When studying coins, the three basic points to be noted are date, provenance, and identification of the images on the front (obverse) and back (reverse) sides of the coins. Dating can usually be established by the image of an emperor or Hellenistic monarch on the obverse of coins. If these images are not present, sometimes the figure on the obverse is known to have been common at a particular time in a certain area, such as Athens being represented by an owl and Epidauros an image of Asclepius. The original dating of these coins would have been made through careful study of the stratigraphy and their relationships to pottery (Chapter 2).

Although coins have a monetary value and are important for studying trade and economy, they also have names and images inscribed on them that inform us about particular events, deities, objects, or structures that represent the places where the coins were minted. In some respects, they help in both reinforcing and shaping an identity of a city state, province, or people by displaying something they deemed important to their region. In some instances, coins display medical imagery that can help us to identify how those living in certain areas wanted to be recognized for their healing activities and/or pharmaceutical ingredients.

Sometimes the coins depict aspects of localized versions of myths associated with gods. For example, coins from Epidauros, dating to the period of Antoninus Pius, whose image is located on the obverse, depicts a cypress tree and a shepherd standing with a goat that is suckling the infant deity (Penn 1994: 16; Paus., 2.26–35). Another example is a medallion minted during the rule of Antoninus Pius which shows Asclepius' arrival Rome. The worship of Asclepius was officially introduced to Rome sometime after 298 BC, when Rome was inflicted with a plague. To ask for help, the Romans sent diplomats to Epidauros, who returned with the sacred snakes from the sanctuary. These were placed on an island in the Tiber originally known for the worship of the god Jupiter. A temple was eventually constructed and dedicated to Asclepius (Livy, *Ab Urbe Condita* 10.47.7; Ovid, *Met.* 15.626–87). The reverse of the particular medallion shows the river god Tiber welcoming a galley with the serpent on its bough. Behind this is an island with a temple and a tree (Penn 1994: 37–8). Here, we see a medical event, deity, and sanctuary important for the depiction of regional identity.

Natural resources were also significant indicators of regional associations and are found depicted on coins. Silphium was a medicinal panacea that only grew in Cyrenaica, where the coins with images of the plant were minted, and was discussed by many ancient writers from the Greco-Roman world (Dioscorides, *Materia Medica* 3.94; Pliny, *HN* 22.38.49; Penn 1994: 79–83). According to Theophrastus (*Hist. Pl.* 6.3.370), the plant was similar to celery. The image on the coin is not only important for regional identity, but because the plant no longer survives, it can provide archaeobotanists with a representation of how it may have looked.

Images placed in private quarters would not have been viewed by a large majority of people. Thus, it needs to be asked if the images signify anything about the person who lived in the space. For example, a Roman fresco of Iapyx, the doctor who treated the Roman hero Aeneas, discussed below, was painted on an interior wall of a probable private home in Pompeii known as the Casa di Sirico, located in area 7 of the city (Fig. 6). It should be asked if there is any surviving information from the house that might indicate the profession of the occupants. One might assume that a medical scene would belong to a doctor. However, this conclusion is questionable. The fresco is not located in a house that had medical tools, as noted by a comparison to Bliquez's (1994) catalogue of medical tools found in Pompeii. Medical objects are one example of the type of small finds that tend to be used as evidence to ascertain the profession of the occupants of other houses in Pompeii. A painting, and even medical tools for that matter, cannot provide us with definitive proof of the occupant's livelihood. It is possible that the scene was significant for another reason, or that the artist was given the freedom to paint a story which they knew well. We also need to ask if the room in which it was placed was in a public or private space in the home. If it was public, it might say something about how an individual wished to be thought of, or it may represent their likes or dislikes.

4.5.2 Ekphrasis

The term ekphrasis refers to the comparison of any form of art that is copied or described in another medium, be it real or imaginative. For example, the shield of Achilles is described in great detail in book 18 of the *Iliad*, and many commentators have used this passage to support their conceptions about Greek *techne*.

Hunt (2005) argues that ekphrasis can also be used to identify scenes painted in art rather than identifying a specific work of art. To illustrate his point, he compares the fresco of Aeneas found at the Casa di Sirico (Fig. 6) with Virgil's description of the wounded Aeneas in book twelve of the *Aeneid*. The painting shows a man injured in the leg leaning on his spear and on a boy. A person, probably a doctor, is kneeling by the man's injured leg, trying to pull something out of his leg with what appears to be a pair of iron forceps. Behind the standing man is a female, likely a goddess, holding red flowers. The image has been identified as Aeneas having a spearhead removed from his thigh by the doctor Iapyx with the help of the goddess Venus and his son, Ascanius. In the poem by Virgil (*Aeneid* 12, 383–440), the ensuing description is given: Aeneas is helped by his son while leaning on his spear for support. Iapyx tries to use herbs to remove the missile but fails. He then pulls and tugs at the missile with forceps. But this fails as well. Then Venus appears, though Iapyx is ignorant of her presence. She causes the doctor to think of and use Cretan dittany to cure Aeneas. Cretan dittany was a plant with downy leaves and scarlet flowers.

The fresco dates to the time in which Virgil lived, so it is likely that the story was commonly known in Italy, at least. However, even if Hunt's analysis is convincing, other questions should be asked about its context, as described in the previous section.

4.5.3 Representations of Medical Practitioners and Tools

What did doctors actually look like in the ancient world? We imagine doctors wearing a white coat or, if they are a surgeon, green or blue scrubs. Both are commonly seen with a stethoscope worn around their necks, especially

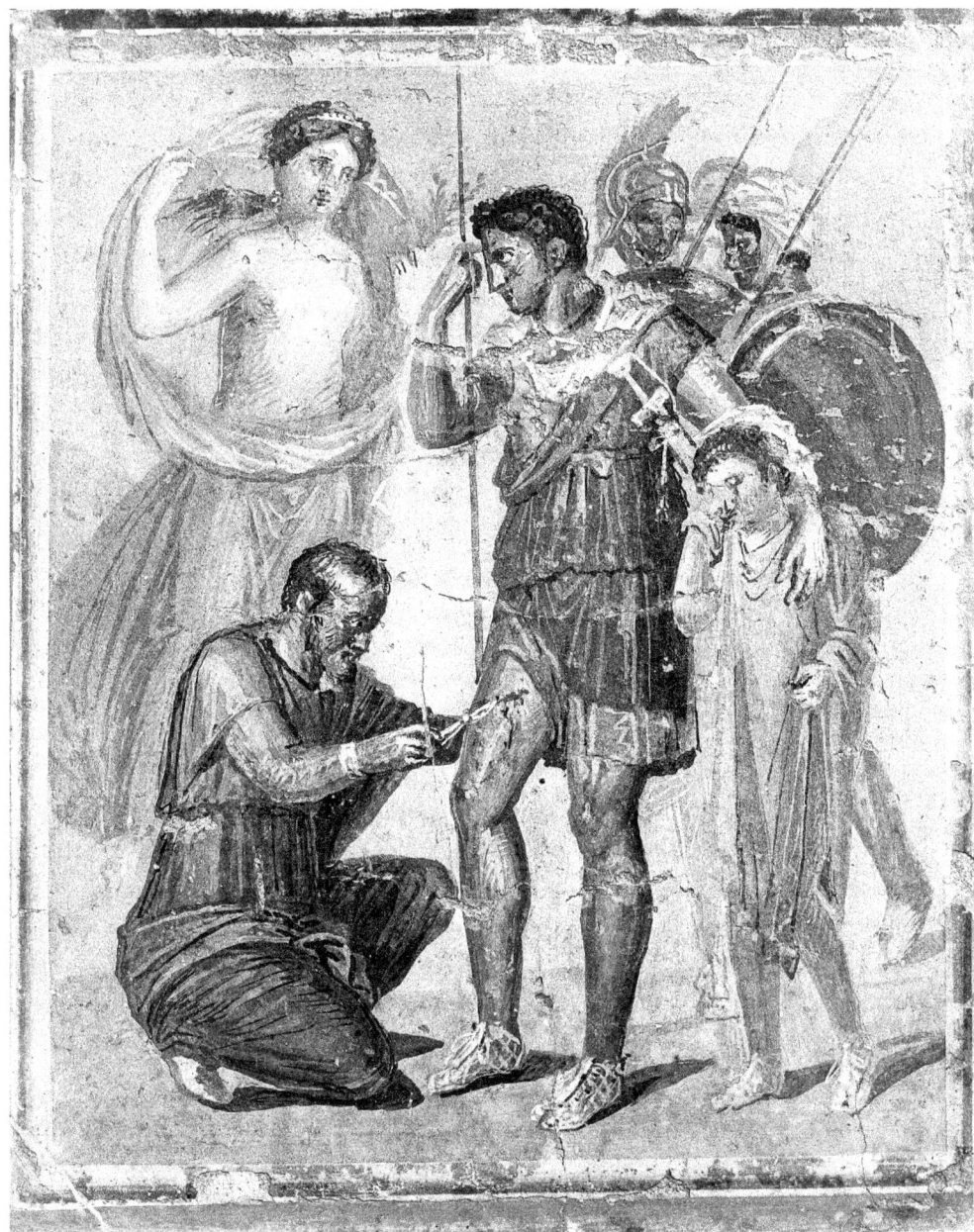

6. Roman fresco painting of the doctor Iapyx treating Aeneas, Casa di Sirico, Pompeii, first century AD. Courtesy of the Wellcome Library, London.

in the media. Our expectations of a doctor's appearance and attributes are influenced by how we see them both in their places of work and in the media. So even though doctors do not always wear stethoscopes or white coats, we have expectations of how a doctor should appear in terms of clothing and material objects, and may become suspicious if they are not seen with these items in a context when they are practicing medicine. It is, therefore, conceivable that there may have been particular "signs" that might have indicated someone was a doctor by the representation of a "standardized" outfit or medical tool. The Hippocratic writers of *On Decorum* (8, 12), the *Canon*, and *Physician* (1), state that a doctor should have a good appearance and be respectful of their patients, but they do not say if a medic should wear certain clothes, only that they should be clean and have tools and unguents available for performing their art.

By examining the images of medical treatment, we can gain some insights into how doctors might have looked. Besides the image of Iapyx (Fig. 6), there are a few other representations of doctors that exist. One is found on a Greek pottery painting, showing the doctor treating patients (Fig. 7). A depiction of a midwife exists on a Roman relief sculpture from Ostia (Fig. 8). The identification of these two people as a doctor and a midwife are plausible interpretations because of what they are doing and how they are using the objects depicted. The first figure shows the doctor with a queue of patients who are easily identifiable by their staffs, bandages, and bodily conditions. Cupping vessels are also depicted above the head of the doctor, and he is seen performing a treatment. A cupping vessel is a rounded, hollow object with a single opening that is placed over the diseased area of the body to draw out blood, pus, or an infected humour. In the Greco-Roman era, they were usually made of bronze. A burning piece of cloth was placed in it to create suction when it was placed on the body. The latter figure shows the midwife's chair, and she is performing her tasks in the same manner as Soranus describes in his *Gynaecology* (2.3–4).

Not all representations of possible healers from the ancient world are as easily identifiable. One from Trajan's Column, a commemorative monument found in Rome venerating the emperor's campaigns in Dacia, depicts a wounded soldier being helped by a person in Roman armour. It is often argued that the helper is a *capsarius*, someone who was responsible for bandaging the injured (Davies 1969b: 84; Jackson 1988: 132; Wilmanns 1995: 135). Scarborough (1968: 254), however, maintains that the image is a soldier rather than a practitioner because the person is wearing armour. He supports this argument with a reference to Dionysius of Halicarnassus (9.50.5), who reported that soldiers sometimes bandaged themselves to avoid active duty. Of course, a counterargument can be made that one could probably expect anyone helping soldiers in the middle of a battle, including doctors or the *capsarius*, to wear armour to protect themselves from injury. Wilmanns (1995: 135) disagrees with Scarborough and says that *capsarii* were so commonly known that anyone would have recognized one on the column. However,

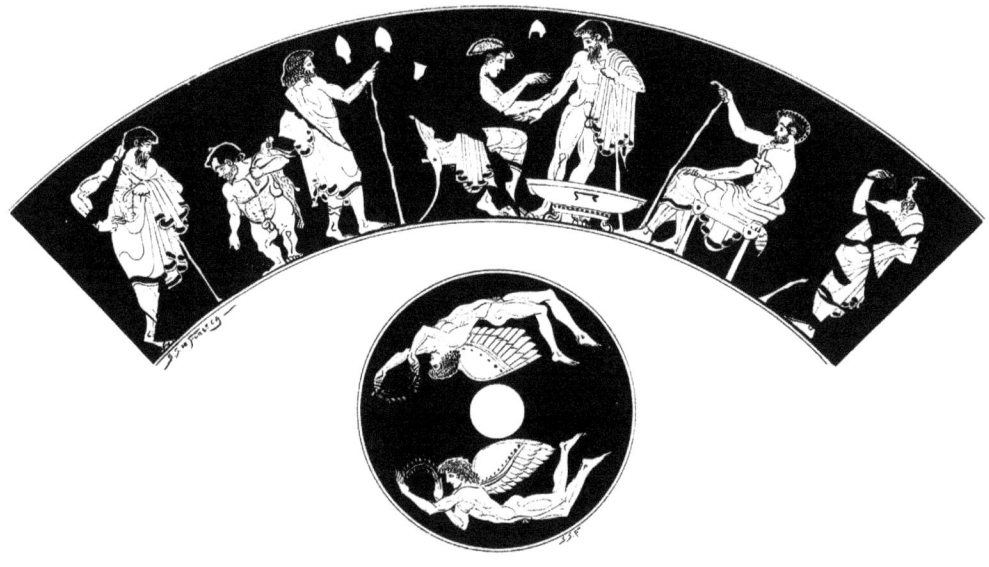

UNE CLINIQUE GRECQUE AU Ve SIÈCLE.
(Vase attique de la collection Peytel).

7. Drawing of a fifth century BC aryballos depicting a doctor or surgeon treating a patient. Notice the cupping vessels above the doctor. Courtesy of the Wellcome Library, London.

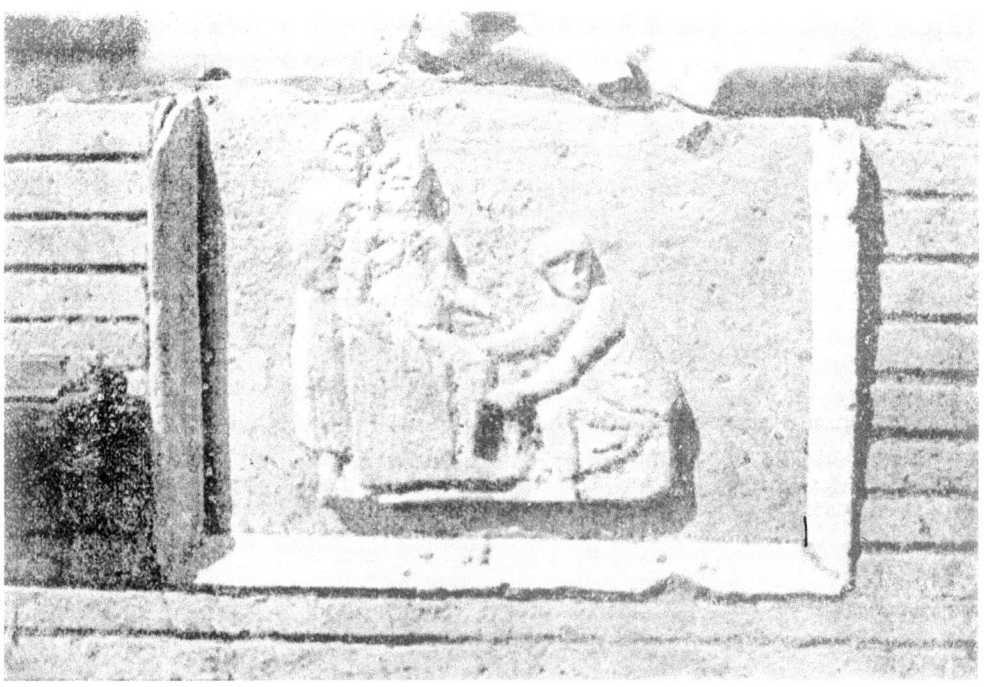

8. Roman relief from Ostia of a midwife, parturient, and the midwife's helper. Courtesy of the Wellcome Library, London.

this assumes there was a medical service waiting along the "sidelines" of a battle, and this might not have existed. This image creates an intriguing problem because it shows that there are sometimes difficulties in identifying the exact role a person held. All that can be said is that some form of help was probably available to the soldiers, but there are no particular signs that indicate this person was definitely a *capsarius*.

Another image is from a funerary stele found in Metz in Gallia Belgica, which has a relief sculpture of a standing female wearing a draped cloak. The word *medica* is inscribed on the monument (*CIL* XIII. 4334; Gummerus 1932: no. 2562). The inscription lets us know who she was, but there is nothing indicated in the relief sculpture that signals her out as being a healer, unless something was painted on her that no longer exists. The point here is that doctors might not have worn anything which may have distinguished them from non-doctors.

It is possible that rather than articles of clothing, certain objects were sometimes used to identify the role of doctors. Although depictions of medical tools are rare, when they are shown, cupping vessels appear quite regularly in comparison to other objects (Figs. 3 and 7). Depictions of the cupping vessels are widespread and found on a variety of Greek and Roman remains from vase paintings, coins, and funerary reliefs that were visible to the public. (To recall a point made above, in societies with low literacy rates, the image of the tool might have advertised the role of the person with whom they were associated.) Cupping, wet and dry, was commonly mentioned in medical texts, and it was the one medical tool specifically created to help balance the humours. In some respects, this object might have been like the modern stethoscope, and acted as a symbol of a doctor who was familiar with humoral medicine.

The images of medical tools are also useful for identifying instruments that are not completely preserved, as is often the case with scalpels. Bronze scalpel handles are a fairly common medical find, but their steel blades have almost always rusted away over time. In this respect, images can provide a better account of the medical tool, since texts rarely give detailed descriptions about the entire scalpel and the variety of blades.

4.5.4 Can Medical Conditions be Identified on Images?

In some instances, archaeologists and medical historians have attempted to use imagery to identify diseases and bodily conditions someone might have suffered during their lifetime. Images of people with debilitating conditions tend to be found on statuettes and votive body parts. Statuettes are smaller, usually less refined, versions of statues. Their original composition was usually terracotta, wood, gold, ivory, bronze, or bone. They are often representations of gods found in households and sanctuaries. In this section, we will consider only the statuettes that show signs of disease.

In the ancient world, ugly and scary images, known as grotesques, could act as apotropaic figures to ward off evil and illness, though they could also have been regarded as comical, given that there were variant views in the past about people with disabilities (Garland 1995: 108–11). As with many of the objects of archaeological concern, the majority of these statuettes do not have a context, and so their exact purposes cannot always be determined. Rather than trying to establish their purposes, the deformities depicted on the figures have been of interest to some archaeologists and medical doctors. In some cases, they have tried to identify the medical condition of the figure. Garland (1995: 117) has noted that signs of gibbosity (hunchback) are sometimes indicated, and Grmek (1988: 58–60) has argued that certain spinal deformations can be clearly identified by the manner in which the spine protrudes from the back of the person depicted, along with the curvature of the spine and shoulders. Nonetheless, it must be remembered that even the medical condition might not be clearly depicted, and the condition represented may not have been understood in the past as it is in the present (see Chapter 7 for a discussion on retrospective diagnosis).

In the case of votives, there are sometimes suggestions that a disease might be identified on the object itself (e.g. Wells 1985). Penn (1994: 96–7) also attempts to find disease and bodily conditions on coins, particularly acromegaly (gigantism) for the emperor Maximinus I. Both are careful to say that their suggestions are speculative. Indeed, in some cases, the disfigurements found on votives and coins might have been formed by mistakes in the manufacturing process. It is, for the most part, impossible to determine an ailment from a votive offering, and care must always be taken when reading about scholarly interpretations of diseases.

Being aware of these difficulties, a more appropriate manner of studying these images is to consider them in terms of disease location (*locus affectus*). Hughes (2008) has recently argued for the possibility that votives can be examined in regards to how people thought of the location of diseases in and on their bodies. There are some votives that depict people pointing to areas of their bodies that may be afflicted. This, along with votives of single body parts, might be a metaphor for conceptions of bodily fragmentation. In comparison to textual sources, Hughes maintains that votives may be "read" in terms of how the ill person envisioned the afflicted body part as being separate from the rest of the healthy body. Thus, healing the afflicted part could be seen as a symbol of returning the entire body to its healthy and complete condition. This is an interesting approach because she does not try to identify particular diseases, but only the location of the disease. The *locus affectus* (e.g. McDonald 2012) was significant in ancient medical literature, and Hughes demonstrates that it is pervasive in public conceptions. Had just the literature been examined, we would not be able to determine if this idea was widespread. Yet, the archaeological remains of images have shown that this was highly likely.

4.5.5 Medical Procedures

Some medical images can be examined for evidence of how surgical treatments might have been performed. The works of Soranus and Celsus sometimes provide descriptions of how procedures were to be executed by midwives and doctors. Yet, in most cases, the descriptions in medical literature, if given at all, are vague. Therefore, pictures can be of greater value than literature when attempting to reconstruct a doctor's surgery, their use of implements, and procedures.

In the modern West, we are familiar with the administering of medical treatments to a patient when he or she is lying or sitting down, with the doctor standing or sitting over him or her. Modern doctor's surgeries and operating theatres are designed to facilitate these procedures. They are well lit and provide a raised place for the patient to lay, with space allotted for the doctor or surgeon to move around the bed or reclining chair. However, in the ancient world, indoor lighting would not have been strong. Because the ability to see the part of the body being treated is one of the most important aspects for performing surgery, doctors would have had to position themselves and the afflicted body part near a good source of light, and this means that they may have had to work outside. It also means that the patient might have had to stand or sit in a particular position for the doctor to treat the patient to the best of his or her ability. Patients are frequently depicted as standing, while the doctor as sitting, kneeling, or standing (e.g. Figs. 3, 6–8). As shown in Figure 6, the doctor Iapyx was kneeling while Aeneas stood. In a Greek pottery painting (Fig. 7), we see the doctor sitting, while most of the patients stand in a queue to be treated. On a relief sculpture from Gallia Belgica, a doctor is shown standing at eye level with a patient while possibly treating the patient's eye (*CIL* XIII: 4668; Gummerus 1932: 91). On the other hand, in the case of childbirth, the midwife is depicted kneeling in front of the parturient (Fig. 8). The parturient is seated on a birthing stool, with a helper standing behind her. In this instance, the relief sculpture matches textual evidence. Soranus gives a thorough account of how the chair was supposed to look and how the patient, midwife, and her helper were to be positioned. The chair is described as having arms on the side and a hole in the centre of the seat to assist the midwife (*Gyn.* 2.3–4).

4.5.6 Body Type

Ubiquitous to the study of ancient art is the concept of the high classical period, Polyklitan idealized body. The fifth-century sculptor, Polyklitos, wrote a work entitled the *Canon* that explained how to create a perfectly proportioned body in sculpture, as seen in his work the *Doryphoros* or "spear bearer" (e.g. Diels 1914: 14–15; Tobin 1975). This statue is one of the main works studied by students of classical art for its style and historical context. Because of its idealized body type, it is also one of the main sculptures against which other fifth-century and later Greek and Roman representations of the human body are measured.

Moving beyond comparisons for stylistic technique, sculptures of this sort can be juxtaposed with ancient medical treatises. For example, a number of the Hippocratic medical treatises describe the healthy body as having balanced humours. The perfect form of the *Doryphoros'* external body, which has symmetrical features, may in fact share a relationship to the perfect balance of the humours. One can perhaps argue that there is a direct correspondence between the perfect balance of humours and the ideal appearance of such a person with this balance. A perfectly healthy person was in some sense physically beautiful.

Another instance of using images and texts together productively can be found in a comparison of the Roman imperial sculpture of Augustus Prima Porta and a description of him in Suetonius' *The Twelve Caesars*. This statue shows Augustus wearing a military breastplate and standing in the same position of the *Doryphoros*. He has a symmetrical body, is muscular, appears young, has perfect posture, and is ideally healthy. However, Suetonius' description of Augustus (*Aug.* 79–82) is far from ideal. Although we should always be suspect of Suetonius because he was writing a century after Augustus was alive and is prone to exaggeration, the contrast between the text and the sculpture is interesting and may be informative of how the Romans envisioned an ideal, healthy body fit for a leader. According to Suetonius, Augustus was perfectly proportioned, but he suffered from weak vision in his left eye and a weak left hip. He was covered with birthmarks, had ringworm, and his teeth were wide apart and poorly kept. Even if Suetonius was exaggerating, by the time Augustus would have become emperor, he would have been older, most likely had wrinkles, and may not have had such an idealized form. As in the example of the perfect balance of humours mentioned above, there seems to be a correspondence between health and appearance. In this case, good health and beautiful appearance correspond, but in addition, what is implied is that these are the result of Augustus' political virtue – or what is captured in the Greek concept of *kalos kai agathos* (beautiful and good). A good person was a beautiful, balanced, and healthy person.

It is not only significant historical characters who can be the subject of such comparisons. Images of soldiers are common on public monuments, and they are shown as strong and healthy. Their imagery is comparable to textual descriptions of soldiers as found, for instance, in Vegetius. He stated that a recruiting officer should look for someone with "alert eyes, straight neck, broad chest, muscular shoulders, strong arms, long fingers, small stomach, slender buttocks, and firm calves and feet without surplus fat" (*de Mil.* 1.6). Vegetius wrote sometime between the late fourth and mid-fifth centuries AD, and his accounts of military life were borrowed from earlier imperial Roman writers. He also wrote a book on animal medicine, so had some veterinary/ medical knowledge (Milner 1996: xxxi; xxxvii–xli). His descriptions of a healthy soldier could have been informed by both the historical texts he used and the animal medicine he practiced. However, it is also quite probable that his descriptions of a well-proportioned and strong body might have been influenced by what he saw depicted on the public monuments. Hence, visual representations might also have influenced medical writers' perceptions of bodily health. It would be odd to think that the two sources were not related in public perception, each informing the other. Taken together, they could represent more commonly held perceptions of health at the time.

In comparison to the ideal body, images also exist of those we would con-sider to be disabled, both physically and socially (in respects to drunkenness and age). These representations should not only be compared to their histori-cal context but also their social and medical context in order to see how those who were less than ideal were understood. Dasen (1988, 1993) has written on the representation of dwarfs and shows that they were sometimes seen as comic figures. More recently, she has argued that children all have dwarf-like qualities (2008). Yet, these images are far less common on public monuments. Rather, they are usually found as small figurines and on pottery painting. They were likely intended for private use, perhaps as something for comic value or as apotropaic figures to protect the owner. A leader would not be repre-sented this way in public art, at least as far as we are aware. Even the emperor Claudius, who was commonly known to be lame, was depicted in the guise of the god Jupiter, with a thoughtful, though not aged, face and idealized body.

As with Augustus, it seems the public image of Claudius involves an identity between idealized appearance and fittingness to rule.

4.5.7 Regional Attributes of Healing Deities

There are not many surviving images related directly to medicine in the Greco-Roman period. However, of those that do exist, a number of them are of healing deities. They are found in a variety of media, such as inscriptions, coins, and statues. The majority that have been identified are of the god Asclepius (Fig. 4). Sometimes he is depicted with his daughter Hygieia (e.g. Jackson 1988: 171, fig. 46). Depictions of Asclepius have been found frequently in the Greek and Roman archaeological record, indicating that he was well known. This frequency, however, does not mean he was perceived and depicted in the same manner.

Indeed, the Greeks and Romans interacted with many groups of people, and there exists ample evidence for religious syncretism between indigenous deities and the Olympian gods (e.g. Green 1992; Webster 1996, 1997a, 1997b; Wells 1999: 163–9). However, the names of indigenous deities worshipped in areas before Greek or Roman contact was made are only known about after Greco-Roman occupation. This is because the names of local deities were recorded only in Greek or Latin. Likewise, figures of indigenous deities did not exist in some places until after colonization. So even the artistic styles were influenced by Greek and Roman practices. Notwithstanding this influence, the indigenous population may have envisioned their deities differently than represented artistically.

The sanctuary at Hochscheid, Germany, for example, was dedicated to both Apollo Grannius, a syncretic deity, and Sirona, a local goddess (Cüppers 1990: 389–91). The gods were identified through inscriptions stating their names (*AE* 1941: 00089). A pair of relief sculptures of the two was found in the *cella* of the sanctuary. They were also identified as both Apollo Grannius and Sirona by their attributes. Apollo Grannius survives in fragmentary form, and he holds a cithara and has his hand on a griffin. The griffin is commonly associated with the god in the Mosel valley and the Rhineland down to Baden Baden. The image of Sirona, on the other hand, is almost complete. As a goddess, she was not well known outside of the region, but she is depicted similarly to the goddess Hygieia, shown with a snake coiled around her left arm. Her other attributes include a bowl of eggs (or so they have been identified as such), and she wears a diadem with a star, supposedly associated with her name, which is thought to have meant "star" (Woolf 2003: 146). It is only the inscribed name that lets us know who she is (Woolf 2003: 147). Interestingly, in this region, it was common for a male god with a Roman name or hybrid Roman name to be paired with an indigenous goddess (Woolf 2003: 147; see also Webster 1997a). Woolf notes that it is curious that she is not depicted with Asclepius, as her association with Apollo does not make sense in terms of Greco-Roman iconography. However, he argues that "[t]he images seem to have worked by themselves, not by virtue of some (well-hidden) master text to which they referred" (Woolf 2003: 148). According to him, the provincial statues must have been seen not for their narrative purposes but as cult statues. The local population would have learnt to recognize them through their attributes. The introduction of statues to the provinces meant that the indigenous populations had to view their own deities through a Roman lens (Elsner 1995).

Rather than fully adopting the worship of the healing deities found in Greece and Rome, here the images inform us that there was a mixing of practices and beliefs. Although it was likely that the god Apollo was introduced into the region through trade with Greece and Rome, he may have been worshipped at this site for his attributes as a healer. Sirona's depiction, similar to that of Hygieia, makes it possible to surmise that she had taken on healing aspects but maintained some of her local characteristics – as, for example, seen in the crown and basket of "eggs". If the objects in the basket are indeed eggs, they might symbolize rebirth or fertility, and perhaps signify that Sirona was also a goddess of childbirth. Obviously, to make such an interpretation, more studies of her imagery need to be made. In any case, this instance demonstrates that images can be informative of a hybridization of healing deities in different regions of the Greco-Roman world.

4.5.8 The Image as an Ingredient to Healing

In the preceding chapter, it was noted that the act of writing was sometimes a necessary component for performing spells that were cast on lead or papyrus. Along with the magical words written on the incantations, images of deities, beasts, and other symbols were drawn on some of the curse tablets. As with the words, the images appear to play an active role in the rituals. In this final section, the concept of an image as an ingredient in healing will be explored.

It has been observed, outside of a medical context, that the use of imagery on grave steles was possibly intended to appease chthonic deities. While the appearance of masonry tools used for measuring and carving stone, such as the *asciae* and *dolabrae*, are commonly thought to have represented the occupations of the deceased as a mason, Susini (1973: 25–6) argues differently. He believes that *asciae* were used like the plough to mark religious boundaries and that by the third century BC, the *asciae* represented the abandonment of the tomb to the chthonic deities. While the plough marked the boundaries of a religious enclosure, the *ascia* marked the boundaries of the inscription (Susini 1973: 25–6). In the light of this observation, it is possible that other objects depicted on graves might have held symbolic functions as well. In any case, the use of imagery on various items appears to have been integral to the objects on which they were represented.

Returning to medicine, images have been found on a number of objects, such as medical instruments and collyrium stamps. In some instances, images of gods and unusual decorative features were made on the handles of medical tools. It is thought that the images of the deities provided added strength to both the doctor performing the treatment and the tools themselves. Some medical tools have been found with handles that look like knotted wood. According to Bliquez (1992), it is quite possible that these are representative of the club of Hercules. Heads of Hercules were sometimes placed on scalpel handles. Although there is little evidence of Hercules being worshipped as a healing deity, he was commonly revered in Rome as a god of strength (Bliquez 1992). Bliquez (1992: 44) notes that the knotty handle is only found on tools used for more difficult procedures – ones that would have required a patient to have a considerable amount of fortitude to endure the procedure. It is also possible that the notty handle represents the staff of Asclepius (Bliquez 1994: 103–4). Or it might indeed have been the intention to invoke both Hercules and Asclepius, adding extra help in both the medical procedure and in personal fortitude. For a similar study relating to surgical knife handles with a mouse and its association with Apollo Smintheus, see Künzl (1983b) and Jackson (1994a).

Collyrium stamps have also been found with decorative images on them that might have been used to imbue the stamp with extra healing power. Some have the caduceus of Asclepius and others have little figures or images of the sun, moon, and warriors. Again it is possible that these acted as symbols of luck that might have helped the patient and doctor and provided extra healing power to the medicines they stamped (Baker 2011: 173–4).

4.6 CONCLUSION

In this chapter, some of the rare images of medical procedures, tools, deities, and doctors were discussed. It was shown that images can be examined in a number of ways that might bring to light concepts of medicine that are rarely described in literature. Therefore, images are an invaluable source of information that help us to articulate the "thousand words" concerning medical practices and beliefs in the past.

CONSIDERATION QUESTIONS

1. Using an anatomical description of an interior body part given by an ancient medical writer (e.g. the heart or uterus), draw what is given in the description. Use your drawing to consider any preconceived notions that might have affected your drawing. Also use your experience to consider difficulties using the texts for descriptions of the body. Consider also how the ancient readers might have envisioned these descriptions and the possible need for drawings to help them understand what they were reading.

2. Whenever examining images in reading, always question what is depicted in them and how they might be used to determine medical practices in the past.

FURTHER READING

Beard, M., and J. Henderson 2001. *Classical Art from Greece to Rome*. Oxford: Oxford University Press.

Boardman, J. 1996 (4th ed.). *Greek Art*. London: Thames and Hudson.

Elsner, J., ed. 1996. *Art and Text in Roman Culture*. Cambridge: Cambridge University Press.

LIMC   *Lexicon Iconographicum Mythologiae Classicae*   Zürich and Munich: Artemis Verlag 1981–1997.

Morphy, H., and M. Perkins 2006. "The Anthropology of Art: A Reflection on its History and Contemporary Practice". In *The Anthropology of Art: A Reader*, H. Morphy and M. Perkins, eds. Oxford: Blackwell, pp. 1–32.

Ramage, N. H., and A. Ramage 2000. *Roman Art*. London: Laurence King.

Various museum catalogues exist for many of the categories listed below.

Numismatic Collections

BMC = 1873–1927. *British Museum Catalogue of Greek Coins*, Vols. 1–29. London: British Museum Press.

BMC RE = Mattingly, H. 1923–75. Coins of the Roman Empire in the British Museum, Vols. 1–6.

Sear, D. R. 1978/9. *Greek Coins and their Values*, Vols. 1–2. London: Seaby.
   1988. *Roman Coins and Their Values*. London: Seaby.

Painted Pottery

CVA   *Corpus Vasorum Antiquorum* http://www.cvaonline.org

Painting

Ling, R. 1991. *Roman Painting*. Cambridge: Cambridge University Press.

Sculpture

Boardman, J. 1978. *Greek Sculpture: The Archaic Period*. London: Thames and Hudson.
   1985. *Greek Sculpture: The Classical Period*. London: Thames and Hudson.

Kleiner, D. E. E. 1992. *Roman Sculpture*. New Haven, CT: Yale University Press.

CHAPTER 5

SMALL FINDS

5.1 INTRODUCTION

The focus of this chapter is the archaeological remains of small finds, such as Greek and Roman medical tools, votive body parts, and medicinal containers. These objects are of great interest to archaeologists because they do not simply serve a single functional purpose, but actively help in communicating, maintaining, and shaping cultural values and relationships between people (e.g. Moore 1982; Hodder 1982b, 2001; Shennan 1996; Tilley 2001). And, in relation to ancient medicine, social rules and activities related to healing and conceptions of health and hygiene can be derived from critical studies of medical artefacts. For example, it was demonstrated in Chapter 2 that modern medical tools are hidden from the patient's view in a doctor's surgery because the sight of even small objects can cause a patient to become anxious. And because the instruments must be treated in certain ways and used in particular manners, this indicates distinct rules of social behaviour that are observed between the doctor and patient. Taken out of a medical context, medical tools will be viewed in other ways that may cause little or no anxiety to the person who comes into contact with them, such as the archaeologist who uses scalpels to separate the Vindolanda tablets described in Chapter 3. Yet, without literary descriptions or direct observation, how does an archaeologist access conceptions about medical objects and rules of behaviour in the past from small finds?

The study of small finds is by no means straightforward. The act of identifying, classifying, cataloguing, and interpreting artefacts requires critical reflection, an awareness of one's own biases in interpretation, and an openness to the possibilities that what we might expect to find may not be supported in the surviving evidence. This last point is, in fact, advantageous. If we are receptive to the prospect of variant outcomes of interpretations, we will be better informed about life in the past than we would be if we were intent on supporting our own assumptions.

To explain the archaeological process of interpreting artefacts, this chapter is divided into four sections. First, the terms "small find" and "artefact" will be clarified in relation to its multivariant meanings. Second, the issues and difficulties involved in artefact classification will be considered. Clarification of such a basic process may seem unnecessary, but because classification is so fundamental, archaeologists need to think about how they are defining and perceiving those artefacts they intend to use in their research. After deciding on a particular set of objects to examine, archaeologists need to collect the information to use in making larger interpretive claims. Section three of this chapter therefore explains the process of gathering and collating material remains that can be used in interpretative analyses. The fourth section follows on from the stage of collecting material by looking at examples which demonstrate how social meanings about medicine can be derived from objects in relation to conceptions of age, exchange, and identity.

5.2 DEFINING THE TERM ARTEFACT

I have chosen to use the term small finds for the title of this chapter because it is more specific than artefact and describes the types of small-scale objects that will be considered herein. Besides the term artefact, small finds are sometimes classified as material culture, but these terms are, in fact, general and can take on various meanings.

The word artefact is derived from the Latin words *ars* and *factum* meaning the skill in joining and making respectively (Caple 2006: 1), indicating that these are objects made and manipulated by humans. Likewise, "material culture" can be described in a similar manner. However, unlike the term artefact, which tends to be associated with objects made in the past, material culture can also be used to describe modern objects. The use of the term culture indicates that various cultural values and beliefs are conveyed in the fabrication and use of the objects. However, anything can be manipulated by humans, so the terms artefact and in some cases material culture also pertain to landscapes, large-scale structures, bodies, and basically everything with which we come into contact (Gamble 2008: 101). In certain respects, these words are what Buchli (2002: 3) refers to as "super-categories" of objects because they take on a variety of definitions and can be interpreted in different ways that are dependent upon the discipline and manner in which the objects are studied (see Berger 2009 and Buchli 2002: 2–19 for an overview). Technically, all of the items discussed in this book fall under the classification of artefact or material culture, so the theories and methods mentioned here are also applicable to them.

Although the terms artefact, material culture, objects, and small finds are commonly used interchangeably, and will be in this chapter, there are certain instances when archaeologists apply precise terminology to distinguish types of objects. For example, a differentiation is sometimes made between different types of artefacts. "Tools" are any objects that are employed as instruments. A statuette, for example, would not be a tool because it is not used to manipulate something physically. Unmodified objects that have been moved from their original location to another, such as taking seashells from the beach as a holiday memento, are given the term "manuport" (Hurcombe 2007: 4–5). These latter two terms – tool and manuport – are mainly used in prehistoric archaeology. It can, however, be argued that these classifications are too prescriptive, as a single Roman medical object can be all of these things. For example, Pliny stated that gem engravers should stare at *smaragdi*, possibly emeralds, and green scarab beetles to refresh their vision (Pliny, *HN* 29.132; 37.62–4). They are artefacts because their meaning is modified; what was a stone or insect is now something that restores vision. They are tools because they are used as an instrument to correct vision. They can also be defined as manuports if the stones and beetles were taken from their original locations to the spaces where the objects were used.

5.3 PROBLEMS OF CLASSIFICATION AND IDENTIFICATION

In order to make sense of the artefacts archaeologists study, they classify them, by function and material, as described in Box One. Although the classification of artefacts might at first seem straightforward and unproblematic, there are inherent biases in the manner in which they are categorized. On one hand, classifications are important because they help us to make sense of the materials with which we are working. Otherwise, we would have one vast category in our artefact catalogues entitled objects or artefacts that would be near impossible to use. How would we find a medical object this way? On the other hand, the classifications are made in terms of modern understandings, and because of this, we tend to assume that their functions would have been the same in the past as they are in the present. For example, a scalpel (Fig. 9) is classified as a surgical tool, which we cannot deny was one of the object's functions. However, it might not have been the only or primary function of the object in the past. It might not have even served a surgical function. One, for example, was found in an archaeological context that suggests it was used for leather working (van Driel-Murray and Gechter 1984: 62). So how does an archaeologist know when objects might have served other functions or did not fit into their ascribed categories?

To answer this question, we need to delve a bit deeper. In the following subsections, we will look at the process of classification and how it is complicated by culturally relative points of views. The anthropological descriptors "etic" and "emic" will help to illustrate how one set of classifications might differ from that made by another society. We will then consider a case study of an object identified as a bracelet in order to show how a system of categorization can lead to "mistakes" or possible misidentifications in artefact classification. Finally, the last subsection presents a brief overview of how developments in the three main stages of theoretical archaeology, described in Chapter 2, affected interpretations and classifications of small finds. From this account, we will see how scholarly theories also affect the manner in which we classify our objects.

5.3.1 Emic and Etic Categories

Artefact classifications found in site reports and catalogues may be an easy means by which we can understand and organize materials, but they are based on modern preconceptions of what an object is and how it should be classified. Classifications are imbued with meanings that might differ from those found in the original societies who used the objects. These distinctions are referred to by anthropologists as emic and etic categories. Emic categories are the views of the object from within the culture which uses it, while etic categories are based on the views of the person studying the society.

The terms emic and etic were taken from linguistic categories. Phon*etics* means the pattern of the language while phon*emics* refers to a word's relationship to other words within a sentence. In etic categories, it is assumed that the classifications are transcultural, or that the same meaning was understood by all. Yet, emic points of view can be quite different and vary between societies (Melas 2001: 140). Praetzellis (2011: 81) provides a clear example of this by referring to classifications of animals. Scientists organize animals according to biological attributes, such as birds having feathers and fish having gills. However, from an emic point of view, animals in Judaism are determined by whether or not they can be eaten in relation to ethical prescriptions made in the Hebrew Bible.

Objects identified as medical tools in the Greco-Roman era suffer from problems of classification made through etic categories. Roman instruments have been divided into two main categories: surgical instruments and toilet

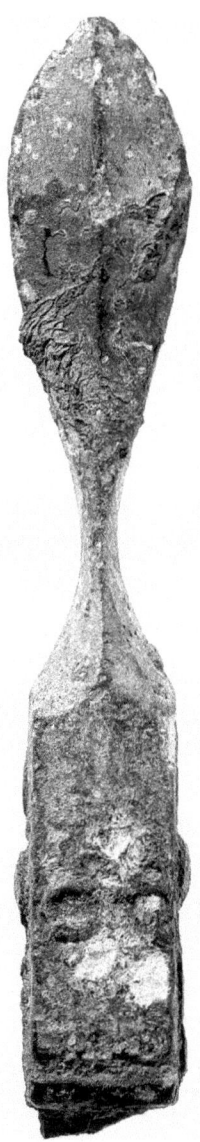

9. Example of a Roman scalpel. Courtesy of the Wellcome Library, London.

instruments. The toilet instruments include ear probes, spoon and spatula probes, and forceps/tweezers. The surgical instruments are scalpels, knives, specula, cataract needles, dental and uvula forceps, and catheters, for example (e.g. Jackson 1990a, 1995; Künzl 1983a, 1996, 2002). These objects were initially identified and placed in these modern categories by archaeologists who compared them to modern surgical implements. The similarity between the modern and ancient objects is striking, so it was a worthwhile comparison to make, especially when archaeologists began trying to make sense of all the materials they were finding in the eighteenth, nineteenth, and early twentieth centuries.

Since the instruments looked like modern surgical tools, archaeologists compared them to their ancient names in Greco-Roman medical texts to determine when and how they might have been used in surgical procedures (Milne 1907). For the most part, the identification of the tools as some form of implement associated with the treatment of the body – be it hygienic and/or surgical – is fairly secure. However, breaking them down into categories of *surgical* and *toilet* instruments is a modern classification that finds no support in the ancient sources. I have argued elsewhere that these typologies of instruments can be misleading (Baker 2004a: 132), since the objects in question can act as surgical instruments, toilet instruments, and tools used for non-medical purposes, such as for painting and for the application of cosmetics. Even the ancient medical texts attest to the multivariant functions of the objects. Quite often, those identified as toilet objects by archaeologists are mentioned in ancient descriptions of surgical procedures. For example, Paul of Aegina (6.13) says that forceps (tweezers) should be used when removing eyelashes in the treatment of opthalmia. The forceps he mentions could simply have been tweezers used in mundane practices of depilation.

There are also problems in classification when instruments are compared to the textual sources. For instance, one of the terms used for a medical probe in Greek is *upaleiptron*. *Ypaleiptron* is used in the Hippocratic works and was derived from the word *upaleiphō*, which means "to spread on thinly" or "to anoint". Hence, an *upaleiptron* was a tool that helped to anoint the patient. We have no illustrations surviving in the ancient texts accompanying these terms, so it is not always possible to make a precise correlation between the different probes that we find in the archaeological record with the names given to them in the texts. Rarely are descriptions of the objects given in the ancient texts. In some instances, we even see terms being used interchangeably, making it even more difficult to determine which instrument the ancient authors were discussing. Sometimes the term *mēlē*, which according to Milne was essentially a probe and not a knife, was mentioned when a surgical procedure would require a knife. Sometimes two terms for one tool were used interchangeably in the same description. Paul of Aegina's (6.8; in Milne 1907: 51–2) description of the inversion of the eyelid uses the terms for both a knife and scalpel.

Thus, these comparative examples, remind us that our etic classifications, although useful to us, might not have been applicable in the Greco-Roman world. Even if the differences are slight, our own biases involved in conceptualizing the function of objects remain.

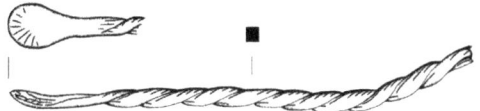

10. Roman "bracelet" from Neatham, Hampshire, England. After Redknapp et al. 1986: 111, nr. 132. Redrawn by Lloyd Bosworth.

5.3.2 Misidentification

Another difficulty with classifications is that some objects, especially those that only survive in fragmentary forms, can be misidentified by archaeologists. For example, an object (Fig. 10) from the Romano-British small town at Neatham, Hampshire, was identified as a "terminal to a bracelet made from twisted bronze rod of square cross-section, with spoon shaped terminal" (Redknap et al. 1986: 111, no. 132). Its end is very similar in shape and size to most objects identified as ligula or ear probes (Fig. 11). It is therefore possible that the bracelet terminal might actually be a ligula. The "bracelet" is broken where the pointed end of the ligula would have been; its opposite end has a slight bend that might have been caused after it was lost. What made me question the original identification of this object as a piece of jewellery was the fact that its end is more like the ligula I have seen. Its handle was also quite straight and not as curved as a bracelet's should be. One of the reasons that this object was most likely not identified as a ligula is because their handles are usually straight, rather than twisted pieces of metal, as seen in Figure 11. However, instrument designs and decorations, particularly on handles, do vary. But since ligula are rarely found with twisted handles, our system of classification has encouraged archaeologists to identify this object as something other than medical.

To see if this object might have had a function besides jewellery, I was able to consider its archaeological context. It was found in a trench belonging to a Roman bath that had exposed the cold plunge bath. Although the object was unstratified within the trench (i.e. we do not know in which stratigraphic layer it was located) and because medical objects are often found in baths, one can argue that the very fact it was in this particular trench lends further support to its toilet/medical function. Consideration of associated artefacts within the trench can also help to support the argument. In this case, a nail cleaner was found in the same trench (Redknap et al. 1986: 111, no. 131).

Although it is plausible that this object was a bracelet, we have a sense from the discussion above of how strongly and unsuspectingly we can be

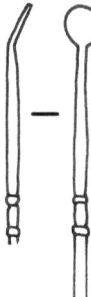

11. Roman ligula. After Jackson 1990: fig. 4.9. Redrawn by
J. Pollard.

affected by modern preconceptions when classifying artefacts. Systems of
classification, in other words, should never be seen as transparent vehicles
for a better understanding. They do in fact aid in understanding the past,
but only if one is aware that the classification is provisional and presupposes
meanings and conceptions that may be biased.

5.3.3 The Influence of Archaeological Theories and the Interpretation of Artefacts

The classification of objects in the archaeological record is also based on the archaeological theories that were prevalent at the time in which objects were collected and studied. In Chapter 2, descriptions of the three main phases of archaeological theory were presented. These were cultural history, processual archaeology, and postprocessual archaeology. The study and classification of small finds, as well as the material culture related to medicine, have been influenced by these theoretical premises.

Beginning with cultural history, when medical artefacts were first collected, they were not only identified as medically related objects, as discussed above, but as being Greek and/or Roman, even if they were found in Germany, Gaul, or Spain. From a cultural historical perspective, the medical objects were seen as having been introduced to these regions by the process of diffusion. This means that social changes only come about when a new group of people move or trade with another group of people. It usually implied that all of the ideas and practices of a colonizing and/or invading group were introduced and adopted by the native inhabitants. This process is traditionally referred to as "Hellenization" and "Romanization" (e.g. Hingley 1996, 2000; Mattingly 1997; Millett 1990a, 1990b; Wallace-Hadrill 2007: 367–70; Zacharia 2008). Hence, medical tools were identified as Greek or Roman objects, and with that came the expectation that they were used and understood in the exact same manner as they were in Greece and Italy.

Object classifications made under the influence of processual archaeology were concerned with various levels of artefact function (Binford 1962: 123–5). On one level, artefacts have a *technomic function*, which to its physical function. This is the function associated with the surrounding environment. The second level is the *sociotechnomic function*, which is related to the object's involvement in social organization. The third is the *ideotechnomic function*, or the function pertaining to the belief systems of the society in which the object is used. Using Roman-period medical tools as an example, we would say that their basic technomic function was their use in surgical procedures for injuries. The object's role as a symbol of a doctor's work is its sociotechnomic function, while its ideotechnomic function would relate to the rules and philosophies of how the tools were used. All of these categories are valid means of interpretation. However, a problem with this approach is that archaeologists originally tended to assume a universal meaning for each object wherever they are found.

In the later 1970s and early 1980s, archaeologists began to realize that there were problems with the idea of these universalizing interpretations. Hodder (1982b) demonstrated in his book *Symbols in Action* that artefacts may have a similar function, but the meanings they held would vary between societies. To understand the functions and meanings of objects, he and others argued that the context and associated artefacts of the object being studied should be noted in order to determine what the object meant to the people who used them.

Not only have these observations led to interesting examinations of material remains, but they have caused archaeologists to be self-reflective about how they are actually making their interpretations. For example, when identifying a cutting object such as a scalpel, an archaeologist will ask how she has arrived at the interpretation that the object is a scalpel used in surgical procedures. She will also consider if there is anything deeply embedded in her manner of thinking that has caused her to make this interpretation. The answer to her questions might be that she arrived at the interpretation because the design of the artefact was similar to modern scalpels. A similarity in form then led her to assume that there was a similarity in function. Without this process of reflection, an archaeologist would be likely to assume that a patient in the past would have had a fear of the scalpel because there generally exists a modern fear of medical objects in Western society.

While it is impossible to rule out all biases and even to know in some foolproof way what biases one is entertaining, there are certain steps the archaeologist can take to enable a broader view of artefacts and their possible range of meanings. These steps include recognizing that every object has a determinant context, and making careful comparisons of designs, materials, colours, and associated artefacts.

5.4 THE PRACTICE OF COLLECTING INFORMATION ABOUT MATERIAL CULTURE

Anyone interested in examining small finds will first need to determine both the types of materials and the questions they wish to ask of them. In this section, the reader will be guided through the steps of collecting artefacts and organizing the information about them with an example of medical tools found in Roman Spain. As with any research, the original questions asked will determine the parameters by which the material is collected and studied.

The archaeologist should also be open to the possibility that what they expect to find might not be supported in the archaeological record. There are cases where scholars set out to "prove" a "fact" about the past before undertaking the research. This is problematic in archaeological research because a specific answer to a question is expected prior to research actually being undertaken. In the worst case, research can simply set out to "verify" the expected answer by ignoring those facts or features which may contradict it. But this is not to say every question is a defeated one. Rather, there are better ways of posing questions that do not tend so strongly towards anticipating a particular answer. For example, a question like "Is there evidence to support the long held idea that there was a uniform system of medical treatment in Roman Spain?" is better than "What is the evidence for a uniform system of medical treatment in Roman Spain?" The former question is more open to different answers, while the latter is already assuming that there was a uniform system of treatment. Although this difference might, at first, seem slight, it can affect how material is studied and collected. With these concerns in mind, let us consider the following example for collecting and studying material in some detail.

5.4.1 Setting the Question and Research Parameters

I wish to know if Roman-style medical practices were adopted by the indigenous inhabitants of the Roman provinces of Hispania after Roman occupation. I am asking this question because there is a general assumption in many archaeological studies of Roman medicine that once the Romans occupied a province, the native population would have become "Romanized". This means that the indigenous inhabitants would have adopted a complete Roman lifestyle, including their medical traditions. This idea is based on little evidence and few, if any, studies of indigenous medical practices. Other areas of provincial Roman research, such as religion, are now challenging the idea of Romanization because the archaeological evidence is demonstrating that the indigenous inhabitants of different provinces had various responses to Roman occupation. In some instances, people adopted new practices and the use of objects; in others, there is clear evidence of a rejection of certain Roman practices; and in still others, there appears to have been a hybridization of practices (e.g. Webster 1997a, 1997b). Thus, I want to know if the medical objects found in Roman-period Spain indicate conformity to Roman medical beliefs and treatments or if they symbolize some other practices.

Having set the question, I now need to decide the time period and objects I wish to study. In this example, I have decided to focus on the period of Roman occupation from the late first century BC to the mid-third century AD. I start out with a broad date range that can be adjusted if necessary. I might find that information only dates to one century and would then need to ask why this is the case.

I also have to decide on the types of objects I wish to consider. In reality, I would examine a range of evidence: literature, epigraphy, and material remains. Yet, in this example, I will explain the small finds that have been identified as surgical tools and keep a record of the surgical tools' associated artefacts. As we saw in the previous section, associate artefacts might produce a pattern of similar objects appearing with the tools. If, for example, a statuette appeared frequently with medical tools, this pattern could indicate that the statuette was integral to ancient treatments. This wider grasp of the context would then allow me to revise my data collection and add or remove material that may or may not be pertinent to my initial question. Once these preliminary parameters are set, I can begin to collect my data.

5.4.2 Collecting Archaeological Data

A database is useful for organizing the data associated with the medical tools I am examining. However, before this is created (actually they are done at the same time, but it is best to describe them separately), I need to find information about the medical tools.

Information about material finds exists in a number of places: archaeological site reports, papers in archaeological journals, and museum lists of special collections, for example. For Spain, I am fortunate that there is a catalogue of Roman medical tools from the province (Borobia Melendo 1988). Catalogues such as these are useful resources for my research. However, they may not include all of the objects from the province, or information necessary for the questions I wish to address in my research. In this case, the archaeological context and associated artefacts are not always discussed in the catalogue. Therefore, I must look elsewhere for this information. In most cases, I will need to consult the original site reports or publications of the artefacts. These should, in theory, be cited in artefact catalogues.

If I decide to peruse site reports to see if there are any medical tools listed that are not described in the catalogues mentioned above, I would have to look under a number of categories. Because most tools are made of copper alloy, iron, or bone, they will be listed under corresponding material headings. If I were to consider vessels used to hold medicines and ointments, I would find them listed under glass and pottery. Stamps used to mark medicines might be placed under inscriptions or perhaps stone artefacts. If organic remains exist, I might even see if some medical tools were made of wood. Albucasis explained that vaginal specula were constructed of boxwood in the

Arabic period (*On Surgery and Instruments* 1.51–2), so there is also a possibility that this material was used in the Roman period.

Certain information should be provided for each object listed in a site report. The artefact should have an artefact number that indicates the site where it was found, the year of excavation, and perhaps the place of excavation on the site. Descriptions of the objects should include details about its size, date, fabric, archaeological provenance, and physical appearance. A photograph or drawing of the object is usually included (Hurcombe 2007: 14–37). Sometimes associated artefacts found with particular objects are mentioned or cross-referenced in these reports. This is commonly done with burials, as seen with the Roman burials found at Mulva in Spain (e.g. Raddatz 1973).

If the reports are incomplete, an archaeologist will have to consult original site notes and even museum collections to see if the information required has been recorded. Sometimes, like the national archaeological museum in Madrid, the medical tools held in the collections will be published (Molina 1981). When the information is unavailable, the curators of individual museums need to be contacted to see if medical objects might be held in their collections. As a case in point, for my PhD thesis, I examined 1,072 instruments; about half of those were either not published, or the publications did not contain all of the information I needed. Consequently, I had to visit a number of museums which contained medical tools along with the original site reports.

In theory, when writing to obtain permission to view museum archives, scholars should be permitted entry. Nonetheless, admittance will vary depending on the regulations of the museum and the condition of the objects. The researcher must also be aware that each museum will have its own system of cataloguing and storing objects. Once the system of cataloguing is explained, the researcher will be given access to the materials. There should be information pertaining to how the materials came into the museum collection. For example, artefacts from an archaeological site are usually acquired by museums as a part of the site archive. Site archives may include all of the artefacts from the excavations, the original site notes and reports, and, in some cases, publications associated with the site and/or objects.

5.4.3 Creating a Database and a Distribution Map

Databases can be formulated in a number of ways: as lists, tables, or catalogues. Most databases of artefacts include information about the type of object, the site, its size, date, publication, museum inventory number, and

TABLE 3. *East Necropolis Medical Burial Number One from Mérida, Spain*

1. Surgical Knife	2. Scalpel	3. Scalpel
Inv. No. NA	Inv. No. NA	Inv. No. NA
Date: NA	Date NA	Date NA
Prov. East Necropolis Medical Tomb One	Prov. East Necropolis Medical Tomb One	Prov. East Necropolis Medical Tomb One
L. NA	L. NA	L. NA
M. CA	M. CA	M. CA
Pub. Floriano 1940/1: 420, no. 1	Pub. Floriano 1940/1: 421	Pub. Floriano 1940/1: 421
4. Ligula	5. Ligula	6. Forceps (tweezers)
Inv. No. NA	Inv. No. NA	Inv. No. NA
Date NA	Date NA	Date NA
Prov. East Necropolis Medical Tomb One	Prov. East Necropolis Medical Tomb One	Prov. East Necropolis Medical Tomb One
L. NA	L. NA	L. NA
M. CA	M. CA	M. CA
Pub. Floriano 1940/1: 424	Pub. Floriano 1940/1: 424	Pub. Floriano 1940/1: 424

Associated artefacts: shears, round pottery container, scale, pottery and glass vessels, and a Claudian coin.

Key: Inv. No., museum inventory number; NA, not available; Prov., provenance within the site; L, length; M, fabric or material the object is made of; Pub., publication; CA, copper alloy.

fabric. Depending on the type of publication, images may not always be needed. In these instances, it is helpful to include generic images of objects to give the reader a sense of how the artefact appeared.

The example of an artefact catalogue given here consists of tables (Tables 3–4). Each table represents a burial that contained medical artefacts from a Roman necropolis at Mérida in Extremadura, Spain. Each box in the table is devoted to one medical tool, and the final box in the table consists of a list of other artefacts found with the medical instruments in the burials. Information from these tables can be used to answer particular issues raised by the archaeologist.

Artefacts can also be compared to other sites. One means of noting where medical artefacts are found is to mark them on a distribution map.

Although the two tables shown are by no means a complete sample, they are intended to demonstrate how an archaeologist might collate her information. By examining and counting information about the objects from tables like this, patterns can emerge. For example, it is noteworthy that many of the instruments in the burials were made of copper alloy (CA). Both burials also contained a coin and objects that might have held medicinal remains, such as glass and pottery vessels. This information can then be compared to other sites and burials in Spain.

If, for example, I wanted to note other sites that contained medical objects in Roman Spain, I could plot these sites on a distribution map (Fig. 12). On

TABLE 4. *East Necropolis Medical Burial Number Two from Mérida, Spain*

1. Scalpel (Octagonal handle) Inv. No. NA Date NA Prov. East Necropolis L. 95 mm M. CA Pub. Alvarez Sáenz de Buruaga and García de Soto 1946: 73, no. 5	2. Forceps (tweezers) with a clasp Inv. No. NA Date NA Prov. East Necropolis L. NA M. CA Pub. Alvarez Sáenz de Buruaga 1945: 5	3 Ligula Inv. No. NA Date NA Prov. East Necropolis L. 140 mm M. CA Pub. Alvarez Sáenz de Buruaga and García de Soto 1946: 73, no. 3
4. Spoon Probe Inv. No. NA Date NA Prov. East Necropolis L. 176 mm M. CA Pub. Alvarez Sáenz de Buruaga and García de Soto 1946: 72, no. 1	5. Rectangular Spatula Probe Inv. No. NA Date NA Prov. East Necropolis L. 176 mm M. CA Pub. Alvarez Sáenz de Buruaga and García de Soto 1946: 72, no. 2	6. Probe (fragment) Inv. No. NA Date NA Prov. East Necropolis L. 116 mm M. CA Pub. Alvarez Sáenz de Buruaga and García de Soto 1946: 75, no. 1
7. Double Ended Olivary Probe Inv. No. NA Date NA Prov. East Necropolis L. 140 mm M. CA Pub. Alvarez Sáenz de Buruaga and García de Soto 1946: 72, no. 2	8. Forceps Inv. No. NA Date NA Prov. East Necropolis L. NA M. CA Pub. Alvarez Sáenz de Buruaga and García de Soto 1946: 73, no. 1	9. Tooth-ended Forceps (tweezers) Inv. No. NA Date NA Prov. East Necropolis L. NA M. CA Pub. Alvarez Sáenz de Buruaga and García de Soto 1946: 73, no. 2

Associated artefacts: fragments of three glass flasks, knife, shears, part of a round box, a coin of Antoninus Pius, and pottery

Key: Inv. No., museum inventory number; NA, not available; Prov., provenance within the site; L, length; M, fabric or material the object is made of; Pub., publication; CA, copper alloy.

the distribution map below, I distinguished two types of sites: those with medical finds and those with burials of medical finds. The distribution map allows me to see if there are any clusters of places with medical information. Of course, a cluster could simply mean that more archaeological excavations have been carried out in particular regions, so again questions need to be asked when examining information of this type. Nonetheless, if it is found that a number of excavations have occurred throughout Spain, and medical objects only appear in particular places, then we need to ask why this is the case.

Once I have decided to compare finds from different sites, I can ask questions to see if the objects were similar or dissimilar in terms of their function, contexts, dates, decorations, materials, size, and associated artefacts. If similarities are found in these comparisons, this is referred to as a pattern. In some

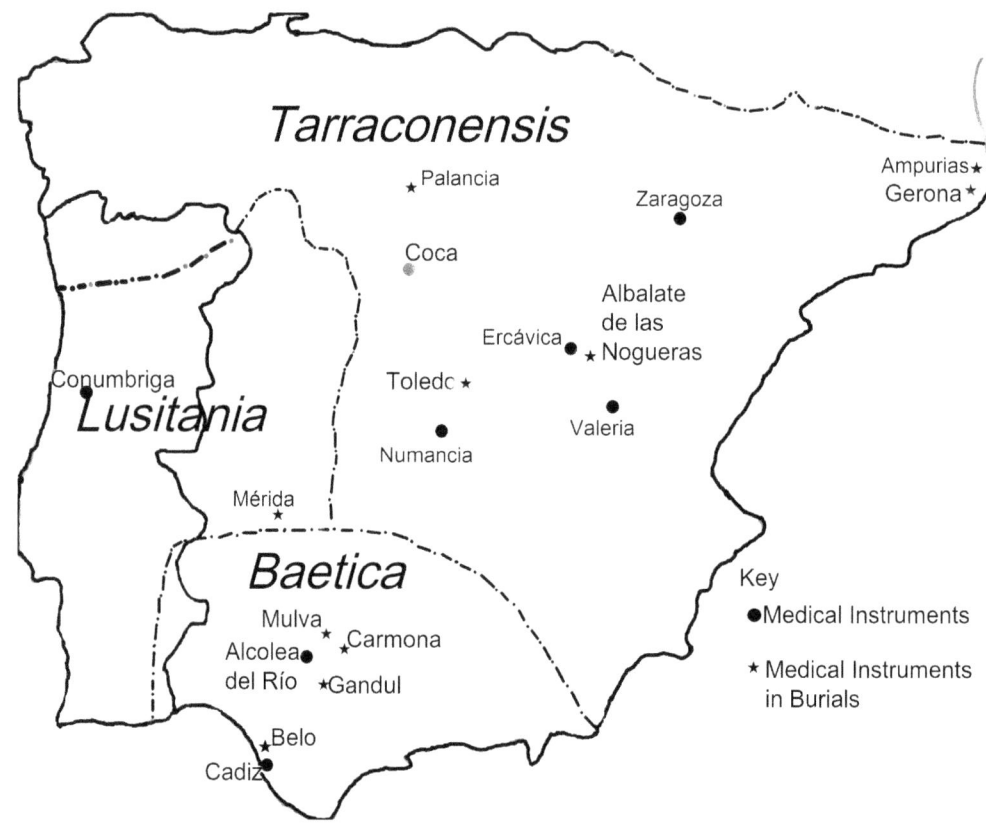

12. Example of a distribution map depicting archaeological sites with finds of medical instruments from Roman Spain, first century AD. Drawing by the author.

cases, the numbers of artefact patterns might be based on a small number of finds, so some archaeologist may wish to use a few statistical tests to see if their data are viable. Although these are sometimes undertaken, statistical tests are always open to question.

Whatever the case may be, catalogues, no matter what format they take, are a tool for helping the archaeologist to sort information that is necessary for developing and answering the questions she wishes to address. Because they are so foundational to archaeological reconstructions of the past, they determine the viability and quality of the next step – the interpretation of data.

5.5 INTERPRETATIONS

Identifying patterns is the precursory step to interpretation of these patterns. In this section, we will look at some examples concerning the types of interpretive questions that can be addressed of material remains. In the first two subsections, we will begin by exploring the kind of information that can be derived, respectively, from objects in relation to their process of manufacture and their deposition in the archaeological record. Then, because objects are not reducible to a strict notion of functionality, the third subsection will examine how conceptions of identity and the exchange of ideas are "located" in artefacts. In the fourth subsection, I will expand the theme of identity to questions of age and sex identification of the tools. The final part concludes with a discussion of the archaeological concept of artefact biographies, which help to show how objects can take on various meanings and functions over time and place.

5.5.1 Fabric, Production, and Identity

As we have seen with processualism, the production of objects has been a prominent interest to archaeologists for quite some time. In some respects, archaeologists are curious about the technologies used in the production of remains and the exchange of materials. In relation to medical objects, there has not been much focus on this aspect of archaeological enquiry. However, the manufacture of objects can inform us about the exchange of medical ideas and practices. It was mentioned in Section 2.3.1 that early interpretations of medical tools found in provincial areas were deemed to have been understood in terms of ideas about Hellenization and Romanization. This meant that when the objects were found in the provinces, they were interpreted as being used and understood in the exact same manner as the Greeks and Romans understood them. However, the concepts of Hellenization and Romanization have been the subject of much scholarly debate in the past two decades. Ultimately, it has been shown that although some of the practices and materials introduced to different regions by the Greeks and Romans were adopted outright, some seem to have been rejected, and many seem to have been adapted to fit local customs and practices. These various reactions have been found in studies of bodily adornment (Carr 2001), art (Wells 1999: 154–6), and religion (Webster 1997a, 1997b). Even the Roman army has been shown to have maintained aspects of their cultural identities, as it consisted of units from different areas of the Roman empire (e.g. Haynes 1999; James 1999, 2002). Gosden and Marshall (1999: 163) argue that the exchange of materials and ideas are bound up in maintaining and constructing social identities when one society encounters another.

Medical tools found in the Roman provinces tend to be fairly similar in design, though there are a few examples where the styles vary considerably to those with which archaeologists are familiar. According to Jones (2002:

90), the designs of artefacts might indicate that there were cultural and social elements afforded to the technological knowledge of production. To put this simply, people may make an object in accordance to their own practices of production and ideas about what materials and styles work best for them. This indicates that although objects are introduced and in certain respects reproduced, the indigenous technologies and ideas are maintained.

In relation to medicine, anthropological studies have shown that societies have strong beliefs about the treatment of their bodies (e.g. Kleinman 1980). When new ideas, concepts, and medicines are introduced to a society, the responses of the indigenous people tend to be no different from those relating to Romanization – that is, there is some combination of rejection, adoption, and adaptation. While the two examples above demonstrated this generally, there is evidence that this also occurs in relation to a people's medical identity (see, e.g., Baker 2004a, 2011; Crummy 2002; Jackson 2007). For example, let us consider a case of technological hybridization which can be found in a set of Roman period medical tools from a cremation burial from Stanway, near Colchester, Britain (Crummy 2002; Jackson 1997, 2007). The burial dates to the mid-first century AD, just after the period of Roman occupation. The tools found in them were similar in appearance to Roman-style medical objects, but they did not completely adhere to the more conventional designs found elsewhere. Moreover, some of the objects were made of iron, rather than the customary copper alloy. Jackson and Crummy argue that the variant designs and materials show that there was an exchange of medical ideas when the Romans invaded the area. Indeed, closer inspection of the material remains makes it clear that Roman ideas were adapted rather than adopted in full.

The same hybridization of medical ideas and technologies of production is found in ritual healing practices in Gaul. For example, the practice of making offerings of votive body parts in healing sanctuaries appears in Gaul after Roman occupation. However, the actual objects deposited are Gallic in design and made of wood rather than clay; they do not look like those found in sanctuaries in Greece and Rome (Webster 1996: 449; Woolf 1998: 217–18). One can therefore surmise that the practice of ritual deposition for healing was adopted, but the materials used were Gallic rather than Roman.

A third example is found with the medical tools from Spain. In my preliminary research, nineteen sites had the remains of medical tools (Fig. 12). Baetica had six, Tarraconensis eleven, and Lusitania two. There are a total number of 298 instruments, with 122 in Baetica, 131 in Tarraconensis, and 45 in Lusitania.

In general, the instruments identified are common types found throughout the Roman Empire: scalpels, forceps, and probes. Yet, the designs of some of the tools were not like those found in other provinces, particularly the scalpels and the collyrium stamps. The reason for this might involve a local preference for a specific style of craftsmanship. One of the three collyrium stamps found in the provinces was unique in design and material, suggesting that although the object was introduced to Spain through Roman contact (or perhaps Gallic given their high numbers in the province), it was not like those found elsewhere in the Empire. Collyrium stamps are usually quadrilateral and made of schist or steatite (Baker 2011; Voinot 1999). Yet, the example is hexagonal (Fig. 13) and dates to the Flavian period (AD 69–98). It was found on the banks of the Rio Salor near Caceres, Extremadura, Spain (Floriano 1940/1: 430–1). It was made of slate local to the region, quite unlike the use of schist and steatite found in Gaul.

Hence, the evidence from Spain demonstrates that although Roman-style medical tools do appear in the province after Roman occupation, they are adapted in design. This adaptation points to variations in medical philosophies and procedures across the Roman empire and indicates the indigenous inhabitants were modifying Greco-Roman medical objects to suit their understandings of health care, technologies in making objects, and perhaps even technologies in holding the objects (see Mauss 1979 [1936] for cultural variations on bodily techniques). In short, if this stamp and the other instruments represent the hybridization of cultural traditions through the medium of newly introduced objects, it also shows that people were maintaining their identities rather than becoming fully "Romanized". To phrase this according to contemporary archaeological theory, one can say that the manner in which objects are consumed contributes to the consumer's identity.

5.5.2 Deposition and Object Meanings

A recent concern in the study of objects is a consideration for how objects acted as metaphors to enforce or perpetuate social rules and practices. Tilley (1999) explained in his book *Metaphor and Material Culture* that the treatment of material culture acts as a metaphor for how we think (see also Tilley 2001, 2002). In other words, the idea here is that archaeologists can access social meanings of finds by considering how they were deposited in the archaeological record. For example, in a modern sense, the manner in which we discard medical tools is fundamentally related to how we treat and use them. A more general illustration of this point can be made in relation to the way in which most objects for us today are disposable: we treat things such as

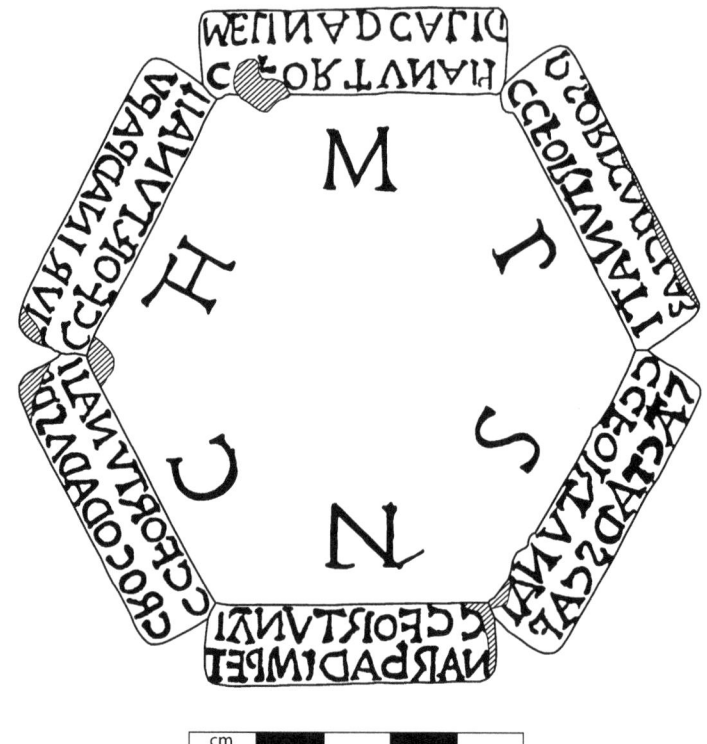

13. Collyrium stamp from Caceres, Spain, late first century AD. After Floriano 1940/1. Redrawn by L. Bosworth. The lettering on each side of the stamp is given in capitals, followed by the complete words in italics. The first letter represents the medicine, the next line is the name of the person who owned the stamp and/or made the medicine (Caius Caccilius Fortunatus), and the third line gives the name of the medicine again and the ailment that it could be used to cure.

[1] M	[3] S	[5] S
CCFORTVNATI	CCFORTVNATI	CCFORTVNATI
MELINADCALIG	STACTADSCAB	CROCADASPR
M(elinum)	*S(tactum*	*C(rocodes*
C(aii C(accilii Fortunati	*C(aii C(accilii Fortunati*	*C(aii C(accilii Fortunati*
Melin(um ad Calig(inem	*Stact(um ad acab(ritiem*	*Crocod(es ad aspr(itudinem*
[2] P	[4] N	[6] TH
CCFORTVNATI	CCFORTVNATI	CCFORTVNATI
PSORICADCLAR	NARDADIMPET	THVRINADAPAV
P(soricum	*N(ardinum*	*Th(urinum*
C(aii C(accilii Fortunati	*C(aii C(accilii Fortunati*	*C(aii C(accilii Fortunati*
Psoric(um ad clar(itatem	*Nard(inum ad impet(igum*	*Thurin(um ad papulas*

plastic bottles, cars, and various forms of computer technology as if they were not intended to last very long. We manufacture, buy, use, and jettison these things knowing full well they are disposable, recyclable, and easily replaceable. With regards to medicine, we believe that used medical tools are unhygienic. So once they are used, the sharp tips are thrown away in special containers that are marked with a biological hazard sign. They will then be incinerated.

Or let us consider an actual archaeological study where the examination of the deposition of Roman medical tools, outside of a burial context, has demonstrated that these tools tended to be deposited in two ways. The first manner of deposition involved those places commonly used for the disposal of refuse, while the second related specifically to places of votive deposition.

Those objects found in rubbish deposits were of especial interest because many of them were in good condition. In fact, the high quality of preservation allowed archaeologists to determine that the objects in question were not "broken" in any sense. It appears that though discarded as rubbish, they could have been reused. From this odd coincidence, I argued that these objects were likely to have been discarded because they may have been perceived as being polluted. It is possible that they were used to treat someone who had died or was seriously ill. If such were the case, the object might have been discarded because it was symbolically associated with the deceased (Baker 2004b). In other instances, medical tools were found in places that were clearly used for votive deposition, such as in rivers and springs. This context suggests that the objects may have been used as offerings to produce good health or a cure (Baker 2004b, 2011). Whatever the case may be – whether in relation to pollution or blessing – one can see from the examples above that deposition is a feature of artefact analysis that provides for a more robust understanding of past social rules and practices.

5.5.3 Sex and Age

Artefacts can also be studied to determine past conceptions of age, sex, and gender. Age and gender are socially constructed concepts. Gender differs from sex in that sex is based upon the biological differences between male and female, while gender is defined according to the roles people play in their societies. So what may be perceived as a masculine role in one society may very well be seen as feminine. Or, as with many indigenous societies, a person – such as a shaman – may be male according to sex but understood as female according to the social role played. This means, of course, the conceptions of gender are much more flexible and variable.

So while sex is defined by anatomy, gender can often be associated with objects. For example, jewellery is commonly perceived as being associated with females while weapons are thought to be associated with men. But because conceptions of gender are so context dependent, it means for the archaeologist that bias is yet again an obstacle to be surmounted. Historically speaking, the identifications mentioned above can be misleading, as they are based on modern biases about the expected behaviours of men and women in modern societies. Indeed, a phenomenon foreign to Western norms is the way in which age is sometimes determinative of gender. In certain societies, children and older adults past childrearing age tend to be amalgamated into a third gender because their social roles are different from those who raise children (for theories on gender and age, see, e.g., Butler 1999; Gero and Conkey 2002; Gilchrist 1994, 1999; Laqueur 1990; Moore 1996; Ortner and Whitehead 1981).

With respect to sex, objects, and medicine, some small finds can be used to consider questions about the treatment of males and females. For example, the shapes of most Roman-style medical implements can be used on anyone. However, catheters and vaginal specula were designed more specifically for the male and female anatomy. The catheters were S-shaped for the male urethra and were longer than the slightly curved and shorter ones used for females. They were tubes that were closed and rounded at the top with a hole on the upper topside. The Roman specula are similar to modern specula, and were made with a rounded priapiscus, the part of the speculum that is inserted into the body, so as not to harm it. The shape of the tools lets us know about people's awareness of male and female anatomy in the past.

Regarding age, we often assume two things about medical implements: (1) smaller instruments would have been used for surgical treatments on children, and (2) tools would have belonged to adults who were doctors. When interpreting the archaeological record, both assumptions can be challenged. First, while tools vary in size, there is no indication that smaller sizes were used on children (or even women). It is possible that tools were designed to fit the doctor's hands, or that sizes were chosen according to the intricacies of the medical procedure. Galen (PA 4–5), for example, explained that he fashioned his own surgical tools out of wax and had them made of bronze, which indicates they might have been designed for the size of his hands. Second, there is at least one instance where a scalpel was found in a burial of a child in Worms, Germany (Künzl 1979/81: 53; 1983a: 78, pl. 53). The context is by no means easy to interpret. Did the scalpel belong to the child? Was this child in training to be a doctor? Or did the scalpel belong to the parents? There are numerous reasons for the tool being placed in the burial, and if it is indicative of the child's status, we might be able to say something about medical education at the time. To determine this, we would need to know the ages of the people buried with the instruments and conduct a comparative examination of similar instances.

5.5.4 The Biography of the Medical Object

In this final section, I would like to call to the reader's attention the idea of an artefact's "use-life" or "biography", though as we will see, there is some debate as to whether the two terms are interchangeable. How objects were understood and used by people — from the time of their manufacture, to the time they were discarded, to the time they became part of the archaeological record — can be said to constitute the biography of an artefact. This is to say that artefacts have a certain kind of autonomous life and can change their meaning over time as people interact with them (see Jones 2002: 83–102). Although it is unlikely that the entire history of an object can be established, noting its context, material, decoration, associated artefacts, and discussion in literature can help determine an artefact's range of meanings and uses.

While the term "biography of an artefact" may be used interchangeably with the term use-life, Gosden and Marshall (1999: 169) and Jones (2002: 84) argue that they do not mean the same thing. According to them, the term use-life is based on a materialist perspective, where materialism concerns specifically the production of the artefact and its material features. Thus, the use-life approach will explain how artefacts were created, how they were used, and how they were discarded. A biography, on the other hand, is broader. It not only considers the use-life of an artefact but how it was involved in constructing and maintaining individual and cultural identities and, of course, how these meanings changed over time.

Akin to the problems we encountered with the classification of artefacts, one can anticipate a similar limitation to the ways in which archaeologists attempt to demarcate different aspects of an artefact's use-life or biography. Gamble (2008: 101–2) and Jones (2002: 83) remark that the manner in which we look for cultural meanings in objects relies on a distinctly modern, Western perspective. Even to speak of separate periods of an artefact's life, in terms of production, consumption, functions, and deposition, is to import concepts that are arguably tainted by the modern market economy and its aim of surplus production. Despite these limitations — after all, we have to begin within our own historical context — this practice of demarcation allows archaeologists to reassemble the multivariant meanings held by an object. In some respects, because these meanings can be held simultaneously, it means an interpretive investigation can both treat a meaning in isolation and view the range of meanings comprehensively – that is, biographically. On this view, it is certainly plausible that while archaeologists tend to focus on one meaning or use of an artefact, or one context in which an artefact is meaningful, there may be multiple meanings and contexts for one artefact. It can therefore be said that an artefact outlives any one archaeological interpretation. Indeed, as we have seen, material culture is complex, and objects hold a variety of meanings and functions for the people who used and came into contact with them. If these meanings were easily decidable, archaeology would have long ago reached its end.

5.6 CONCLUSION

Small finds appear to be anything but small in stature. Because artefacts have multivariant functions and meanings that can change with respect to their social and temporal contexts, the archaeologist is required to undertake critical and reflective steps when considering how she is to approach her research. Objects are not simply representative of social interactions, but are actively involved in constructing them. And this means archaeology does not simply unearth extant objects; from the start, it assumes an interpretive posture guided by the best kinds of questions we can possibly formulate. As we have seen in this chapter, medical tools are perhaps one of the best examples of the complexity involved in archaeological investigation. Modern scientific preconceptions are often nothing but barriers to understanding how different people, with different technologies and notions of health and identity, perceived the meanings and uses of those objects integral to everyday life. The objects are, in this sense, the living representations of a people.

CONSIDERATION QUESTIONS

1. Consider how you feel about medical objects in a modern context. How do you react to them and what do you do with them? Do you think there might have been similarities or differences in the way the Greeks and Romans thought about them? Why might this be?
2. Why is it important to consider all aspects of an object: design, decoration, material, and context? What might these tell us about medical concepts and practices in the past?

FURTHER READING

Undergraduate students reading this list will find that some of the information is in foreign languages. The information is still worth perusing because the bibliography list is easily negotiated and images are contained in some of the texts.

One of the most thorough catalogues of publications for information about medical tools in the Greco-Roman world is the one created by Künzl. It lists an extensive amount of publications that reference medical tools and cross-references them by type, place, context, and material.

Bliquez, Künzl, and Jackson have undertaken a considerable amount of work cataloguing and describing medical instruments. Some of their key works are:

Bliquez, L. 1981a. "An Unidentified Roman Surgical Instrument in Bingen", *Journal of History of Medicine* 36(2): 219–20.

1981b. "Greek and Roman Medicine", *Archaeology* 34(2): 10–17.

1994. *Roman Surgical Instruments and Minor Objects Found in the University of Mississippi*. Göteborg: P. Åström's Förlag.

Bliquez, L., and J. P. Oleson 1994. "The Origins, Early History and Applications of the *Pyoulkos* (syringe)". In *Science et Vie Intellectuelle à Alexandrie*, G. Argoud, ed. Saint-Étienne: Publications de l'Université de Saint-Étienne, pp. 83–103.

Jackson, R. 1990a. "Roman Doctors and their Instruments: Recent Research into Ancient Practice", *Journal of Roman Archaeology* 3: 5–27.

1993. "Roman Medicine: Practitioners and their Practices". In *Aufstieg und Niedergang der Romischen Welt* II 37.1, H. Temporini and W. Haase, eds. Berlin: Walter de Gruyter, pp. 79–100.

1994b. "Styphylagra, Staphylocaustes, Uvulectomy and Haemorrhoidectomy: The Roman Instruments and Operations". In *From Epidauros to Salerno: Symposium Held at the European University Centre for Cultural Heritage, Ravello, April 1990*, A. Krug, ed. Rixensart: Pact Belgium, p. 167–85.

1994c. "The Surgical Instruments, Appliances and Equipment in Celsus' *De Medicina*". In *La Médecine de Celse*, G. Sabbah and J. Mundry, eds. Saint-Étienne: Publications de l'Université Saint-Étienne, pp. 167–209.

1995. "The Composition of Roman Medical *Instrumentaria* as an Indicator of Medical Practice: A Provisional Assessment". In *Ancient Medicine in its Socio-Cultural Context*, Ph. J. van der Eijk, H. F. J. Horstmanshoff, and P. H. Schrijvers, eds. Amsterdam: Rodopi Press, pp. 189–208.

1997. "An Ancient British Medical Kit from Stanway, Essex", *The Lancet* 350(9089): 1471–3.

2002. "Roman Surgery: The Evidence of the Instruments". In *The Archaeology of Medicine Papers Given at the Session of the Annual Conference of the Theoretical Archaeology Group Held at the University of Birmingham on 20 December 1998*, R. Arnott, ed. Oxford: British Archaeological Reports International Series 1046, pp. 87–94.

2005. "Holding on to Health? Bone Surgery and Instrumentation in the Roman Empire". In *Health in Antiquity*, H. King, ed. London: Routledge, pp. 97–119.

2007. "The Surgical Instruments". In *Stanway: An Élite Burial Site at Camulodunum*, P. Crummy, S. Benfield, N. Crummy, V. Rigby, and D. Shimmin, eds. Britannia Monograph Series no. 24. London: Society for the Promotion of Roman Studies, pp. 236–52.

Künzl, E. 1979/81. "Medizinische Instrumente aus dem römischen Altertum in Städtischen Museum Worms", *Der Wormsgau* 13: 49–63.

1982. "Römische Medizin im Spiegel archäologischer Funde", *Archäologie in Deutschland* 1(Jan–März) 14.

1983a. *Medizinische Instrumente aus Sepulkralfunden der römischen Kaiserzeit*. Cologne: Rheinland Verlag GmbH.

1984. "Einige Bemerkungen zu den Herstellern der romischen medizinischen Instrumente", *Alba Regia* 21: 59–65.

1996. "Forschungsbericht zu den antiken medizinischen Instrumenten", in *Aufstieg und Niedergang der Romischen Welt* II 37.3, H. Temporini and W. Haase, eds. Berlin: Walter de Gruyter, pp. 2433–639.

2002. *Medizin in der Antike: aus einer Welt ohne Narkose und Aspirin*. Stuttgart: Konrad Theiss Verlag GmbH.

CHAPTER 6

HEALING SPACES

6.1 INTRODUCTION

In this chapter, we consider how archaeological remains are associated with healing spaces. Because artefacts simply exist neither in a vacuum nor in a space homogenous with our own cultural practices, it is essential for an archaeologist to consider material remains along with the sites mentioned in ancient texts. As we will see, in attempting to understand social rules and meanings, there is a strong interrelation between artefacts and sites. Moreover, we will see by the conclusion of this chapter that, with sites, there is a mutual relation in which a site will reinforce social norms of a people and, conversely, a people will construct sites according to these existing norms.

The first section of this chapter will briefly explain how sites, spaces, and structures related to medicine and healing are identified in the archaeological record. As the reader might have guessed, similar to the problem of cultural bias in the classification of artefacts, we will see how site identification is not a simple task and often suffers from gross assumptions when determining what certain structures may have been and the functions they may have performed. In a previous study of Roman military hospitals (*valetudinaria*), I found that the original archaeological identification could not be securely supported (Baker 2002b, 2004a: 83–114). We will consider this study later, but let it suffice to say here that simply because a building has been identified on a site plan does not mean this identification is certain.

The second and third sections address in some detail how spaces can be investigated as a way of determining social conceptions of health and hygiene in the past. For example, returning to the description of my doctor's surgery mentioned in Chapter 2, it was shown that the layout of the doctor's surgery and the placement of the waiting areas reinforced patterns of behaviour that were significantly linked to modern social rules regarding health care and privacy. Social rules can also be found in the archaeological record through an investigation of surviving spaces. Such an exercise may seem easy enough when investigating a modern space for which we know many of the rules and norms defining it. But the task becomes significantly more difficult when dealing with past cultures for which we know very little, or worse yet, think we know quite well but really do not. Using the example of an *abaton*, or a building used for the practice of incubation at healing sanctuaries, the second section provides a step-by-step guide for formulating critical questions about previously identified structures.

The third section explains some of the anthropological and philosophical theories that have informed archaeological studies of space. We will consider some examples of the types of questions that can be asked about structures and landscapes, in order to see how past conceptions of hygiene and health might have informed the construction of certain civic amenities, such as the supply of water and baths. Conversely, we will examine Roman baths and latrines to show how the layout of these spaces reinforced and informed social rules of modesty that might have affected ancient attitudes towards spaces of treatment.

Finally, the chapter will conclude with a short discussion that compares ancient literature with archaeological sites to see if each type of evidence supports a general representation of what constitutes a salubrious environment in the Greco-Roman world.

6.2 WHAT DOES THE EXTANT LITERATURE TELL US OF ANCIENT HEALING SPACES?

Extant literary and epigraphic evidence from the Greco-Roman world indicates that medical treatments were performed in various places: homes, bedchambers, hospitals, baths, doctors' houses, and healing sanctuaries. People might also have received treatment in shops, or what Harig (1971: 189) and Jackson (1988: 65) refer to as *taberna medica* (medical shops). *Tabernae medicae* are not mentioned in ancient literature, but Harig convincingly argued that there were likely public places in the Roman world where people could receive medical treatment. He bases his interpretation on literary excerpts that mention the Greek *iatreia* (e.g. Plato, *Rep.* 3.405a). *Iatreia* translates to a surgery, or some form of consulting room, which were possibly located in towns and/or markets. When it comes to descriptions of all of these spaces, however, the ancient literature provides few, if any, details about their layouts, amenities, or furnishings. For example, the Roman writer Hyginus provided a description of the location of the *valetudinarium* in the fortification in his *Liber de Munitionibus Castrorum* (4). According to him, the *valetudinarium* should be constructed beyond the *praetorium*, which was either the commanding officer's private quarters or the central section of the camp. He suggested that it should be placed about seventy Roman feet from the *veterinarium* (animal hospital/ shelter) and the *fabrica* (workshop) because this was a quiet location. From this, it is often assumed by archaeologists that all Roman military hospitals were placed in the same area (e.g. von Petrikovitz 1975: 98). However, there is no real evidence to support this conclusion. Hyginus provides no details of size, shape, layout, or amenities within the structure, and his account is the only surviving, "detailed" description.

In regards to descriptions of other healing spaces, comments tend to be equally vague. We are usually told that in order to perform surgical treatment, the two most important features are the availability of good lighting (e.g. Hp, *In the Surgery*, 2–3) and the placement of the sickbed. On the latter, the Hippocratic writer of *Decorum* (15) states

> The bed also must be considered. The season and the kind of illness will make a difference. Some patients are put in breezy spots, others into covered places or underground. Consider also noises and smells, especially the smell of wine. This is distinctly bad and you must shun it or change it. (Jones Trans. 1959)

We have no idea from these statements where the rooms were located, their size, how they were furnished, or how large the bed was. In fact, the two Hippocratic excerpts suggest an inconsistency, rather than standardization, of healing space organization. It seems rather than appealing to a default plan, healing spaces were dependent upon the needs of the doctor and, interestingly, the relationship of the space to humoral balance (see also Rosen 2012 for a discussion of *kline* or sickbed).

In the Greco-Roman medical tradition, one of the fundamental conceptions of health and illness was related to the balance of the four humours (yellow bile, black bile, phlegm, and blood). If someone was ill, his or her humours were perceived to be out of balance. To return the body to its normal and balanced state, the doctor would suggest a treatment of opposites. For example, if someone was suffering from too much black bile, which had the properties of dryness and coldness, the patient would have been placed in a warm area and given warm, moist foods and drinks to return the humours to balance. Admittedly, this is a simplified description of the system, but it provides the reader with the basic details of the medical system described in much of the ancient medical literature (see King

2001; Hp, *Nat. Hom.*). It also supports the idea that the sick were placed in different areas according to their illness, at least if the doctor had been trained in this tradition.

Nonetheless, having just shown that we have no clear descriptions of healing spaces, and that they were likely not standardized, the authors of modern secondary sources and archaeological site guides confidently pinpoint single structures and even rooms for specific healing functions. For example, a hospital is identified at Housesteads Roman fort on Hadrian's Wall (Crow 1995: 50–1), and an *abaton* is indicated on the site plan of Epidauros (Charitonidou 1978: 32–4; Tomlinson 1983: 67–8).

These erroneous, modern classifications of ancient structures and spaces tended to be assigned to buildings in the late nineteenth and early twentieth centuries on the basis of exaggerated interpretations of literary references and/or a minimal amount of archaeological remains. The archaeologists also described these buildings in terms of those things with which they were familiar during their own social setting, such as hospitals having operating theatres and kitchens. In instances such as these, cultural bias can not only lead to gross assumptions but also a blindness to seek evidence to support one's claims (Baker 2002b). This is because what is most familiar to the archaeologist can be taken for granted as a norm. This problem may sound easy enough to remedy, but it is more common than one might think.

Let us consider, for example, the first so-called military hospital (Fig. 14) which was identified at the Roman legionary fortress at Neuss in Germania Inferior. It was designated a hospital because it contained a room with ten medical probes. Four scalpels were found in other rooms of the same structure. A drain was excavated in the building, which could have come from a latrine, but there are no remains of the latrine (Koenen 1904).

The building at Neuss was a courtyard-style structure, though it only survives in part, as noted in Figure 14. The layout of the building had a number of small rooms, thought to be wards, that surrounded the courtyard and were divided by hallways. Once this identification had been made, it set a precedent, and buildings of similar design found in other fortifications were then named hospitals (i.e. Baatz 1970: 8–10; Jackson 1988: 136–7; Majno 1975: 382–96; Nutton 1969: 262–3; von Petrikovitz 1975: 88; Scarborough 1976: 68; Wilmanns 1995: 104–5). Looking at the social context of the archaeologist who studied the structures at Neuss, one sees that the so-called ancient hospital was somewhat similar in plan to German civilian and military hospitals of the seventeenth, eighteenth, and nineteenth centuries (Brat 1966; Jettner 1966: 82, 144–5). It is plausible, then, that the archaeologist's

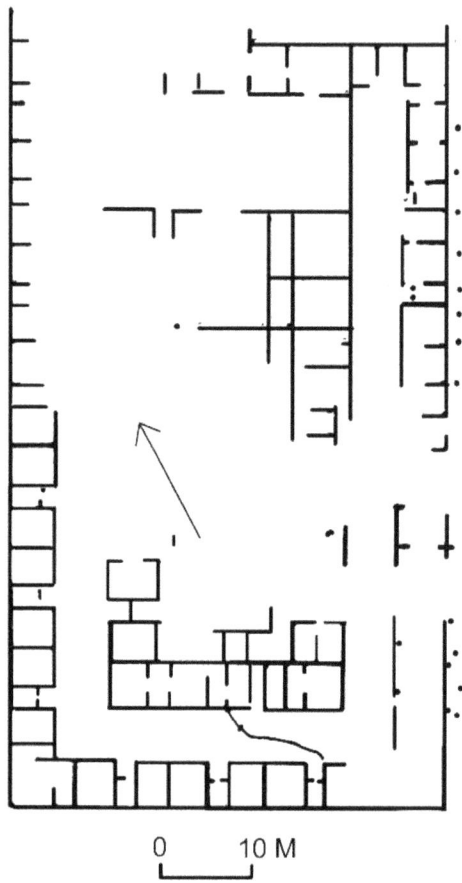

0   10 M

14. So-called hospital from Neuss. After Johnson (1983: 160). Redrawn by the author.

own sense of modern healing spaces contributed to the expectations of how ancient hospitals were designed.

Most scholars unaware of archaeological methods will not think to question original interpretations that tend to set precedents for the wider field of research; this is even a problem within archaeology itself. Questioning long-established opinions can meet with resistance. Reconsideration of past judgements, however, is essential. Accepting older views outright and using them in interpretations can mean that the study one is undertaking may be based on weak foundations (no pun intended). Even when the classifications of structures and spaces seem secure, it is advisable to consider how the original interpretations were arrived at, and if there was enough evidence to support the interpretations at the time they were made. In some cases, the original argument may be validated; in others, there may be cause for reassessment. And this dilemma leads to a further methodological development: how do archaeologists re-evaluate and/or identify sites and structures?

6.3 IDENTIFYING SITES

In this section, the reader will be introduced to the questions archaeologists ask when identifying sites and structures. First, we will begin with some fundamental questions of locating a site and its functions. We will then consider more specific medically related examples that explain how a building identification can be re-evaluated.

6.3.1 Establishing Site Names

One of the fundamental concerns of archaeological excavation is the task of identifying a site's ancient name, in cases of historical or ethnohistorical archaeology, and its function. Sites are referred to by both ancient and modern names, although in some cases, it is impossible to determine the ancient name of a site. In such circumstances, its modern appellation will be used. There are also instances when ancient names have been applied to sites without solid evidence. A good example of this is Troy. Heinrich Schliemann based his identification of the site on his belief that there was an historical Troy. The Bronze Age site he investigated in Hisarlik, Turkey, had no inscriptions. In addition, some of its levels were devastated in the excavations, and this in turn meant the archaeological remains that might have helped to identify its name were destroyed. Nonetheless, the ruins are still referred to as Ilium or Troy. Although archaeologists and historians are aware of "false" designations like this, someone outside of the discipline, who is unacquainted with the difficulties of interpretation, may believe the ancient name applied is secure. So let us consider how archaeologists securely identify the name and function of an ancient site.

The majority of archaeological sites discussed in this chapter have been properly identified, in both their name and functions, through a combination of evidence: inscriptions, discussions in ancient texts, architectural details, and small finds. Even though we can safely say that the healing sanctuary at Epidauros has been properly identified, it is used here to demonstrate where difficulties may lie when archaeologists attempt to determine the name of a site, particularly when they are relying on ancient literature.

When describing his visit to the Asclepion at Epidauros, Pausanias explained how he travelled to the site. He stated, "At Lessa the Argive territory joins that of Epidauros. But before you reach Epidauros itself you will come to the sanctuary of Asclepius" (2.26). He lets the reader know that the sanctuary was outside of the city of Epidauros. However, even given this description, if the remains of both the city and the sanctuary or just one of the sites survived, it would be impossible to determine which site was the sanctuary and which site was the city. This is because Pausanias does not give us distances between the two places, descriptions about their sizes, and any information about whether or not there were smaller settlements located between the two sites. To determine which site was the city and which one was the sanctuary, an archaeologist could begin by asking from which direction did Pausanias approach the city of Epidauros? This would tell us which of the two sites he reached first. Yet, we only have minor details about the direction from which he travelled. He said that he came to Epidauros from Argos after visiting the ruins of Tiryns. At Tiryns, he walked in the seaward direction (Paus. 25.8–9). Although archaeologists have identified the Bronze Age site of Tiryns, we should ask if this was the same site of which Pausanias spoke, and if we know for certain which road Pausanias might have taken when he travelled to Epidauros.

Despite these problems, Pausanias does provide his readers with a useful description of the healing sanctuary. He mentions several structures: the *tholos* or "round house", as he calls it; the stele (*iamata* as we call them) with inscriptions to Asclepius; the theatre; a couple of other sanctuaries; a few temples; a fountain; a stadium; and a dwelling (Paus. 27:3–7). While he never provides a thorough description of any of these structures (nor does he state where they are in relation to one another), the *tholos*, baths, theatre, stadium, and inscriptions have easily recognizable building foundations. However, other sanctuaries and even secular sites within cities contain all of these building types as well. Cities also have sacred areas within them. So identifying an entire site such as Epidauros as a healing sanctuary on a few structures alone is problematic. We can only say, on the basis of the temple foundations, that there were some sacred areas at the site.

Fortunately, we have inscriptions from Epidauros that provide us with evidence for the activities that people took part in at the site, particularly incubation. The god Asclepius is also mentioned on them. However, it also must be determined whether these inscriptions were found in situ or were at least local to the site. There are instances where inscriptions were removed from sites and used as building materials in other places. The quantity of inscriptions dedicated to a certain deity or mentioning a place name found in close proximity to one another will help to confirm the site's name and/or function.

Finally, an archaeologist should also examine the small finds located within an area to try to establish its function(s). Numerous votive offerings were uncovered at the site, which further confirmed its identity as the healing sanctuary. Therefore, when comparing all of the available evidence, we can safely say that it was correctly identified.

When no ancient name for a site can be determined, archaeologists will still attempt to discern the types of activities that took place at a site by considering all of the available evidence. For instance, the function of a Roman-period sanctuary located at Essarois in Burgundy was identified by votive offerings and altars found at the site. An altar was discovered dedicated to the syncretic deity, Apollo Vindonnus. While we have no clear evidence from the inscription what purpose this deity served, we can formulate an idea based upon an understanding of the syncretic nature of the deity and the small finds at the site. Aside from being associated with several qualities, such as prophecy, Apollo was a healer. Vindonnus was local to the region, and may also have been associated with healing. There is some evidence for this: amongst the small finds from the site were numerous votive body parts and bronze plaques of eyes that indicate people visited the place as a healing sanctuary (Detys 1988: 84; Green 1992: 32). To be sure, other types of votives were also recovered that suggest the sanctuary may have been visited for purposes that extended beyond health, but because of the consistency of artefacts types and the syncretic name of the deity, the site is thought to have been a sanctuary.

6.3.3 Identifying Structures

Beyond the primary identification of sites, archaeologists are also concerned with recognizing the functions of buildings and structures they excavate. This is not always an easy task, particularly when buildings only survive in ruins. Structures, like sites, can be modified over time. They can be reconstructed, altered, demolished, or have their function changed over time. The Athenian Parthenon, for example, was originally built as a temple to Athena. It was destroyed during the Persian war in the fifth century BC and rebuilt to celebrate the Athenian victory of the Persians in the same century. Alterations to it were made during the Byzantine period when it became a Christian church dedicated to the Virgin Mary. When Athens was under Ottoman rule, it was used as a mosque and then an ammunition store, at which point it was destroyed. It has now been restored to its mid-fifth-century manifestation and is symbolic of modern Greece – quite different from its original construction when it was a symbol of the Athenian city state.

As mentioned earlier, particular structures or areas within sites were often identified when they were first excavated. Many of these identifications have remained unchanged, without much critical consideration. This is not simply the case with Greco-Roman healing sanctuaries, but is general to archaeological studies. Another problem, particularly in association with classical archaeology, is as Jameson (1990: 93) notes: many building identifications were often derived from literary descriptions rather than from a close consideration of the archaeological materials. Sometimes these identifications are made with "dubious justification", to quote Jameson.

Often, when a structure was identified at one site, it was then compared to buildings with similar foundations at other sites, and the same designation was applied. This is a precarious means of naming buildings for a number of reasons. First, it is possible that original structures were not properly identified. Second, it is made on the foundation alone, usually without an examination of the small finds from the structure. Third, this does not account for regional variations in building use, local concepts of space, the possibility of a structure being multifunctional, and the possibility that its function altered over time. Ascribing a name and single function to a structure without a detailed study prohibits further consideration of what their uses and meanings might have been, and how these could have changed. This was clearly seen with the identification of military *valetudinaria*, and as mentioned earlier, the first so-called hospital identified at Neuss. After these precedents of identification, it was not an unusual practice to excavate only partially those buildings deemed to have similar foundations. Moreover, many of these hastily identified "hospitals" had no medical finds. Indeed, when looking closely at the small finds and remains of these structures, it became apparent that some of them, either in their entirety or in part, might have been used as workshops (Baker 2002b, 2004a).

6.3.3 Step-by-Step Questions to be Addressed When Identifying Buildings: The Case of *Abatons*

This section provides instructions about how archaeologists can question the identity of a structure. This is demonstrated using the example of *abatons*, or incubation halls, which are structures commonly mentioned in studies of Greco-Roman healing sanctuaries and are identified on plans of Asclepia. We are certain that something called an *abaton* existed in ancient Greece and Rome, but as to its appearance and spatial arrangement, we are less certain. As an archaeologist approaching the question of what an *abaton* may have looked like, our first point of access is the existing description in site reports. This process is much like checking the plausibility of another person's translation of a text. Does one agree with the translation and interpretation? As discussed in the previous chapter, when making enquiries of this sort, I should have no prior expectations of the answer I will find. If the evidence supports the identification of *abatons*, then it will be secure, and I can undertake my research on the subject. If the evidence does not support the identification, some re-evaluation is necessary, and it helps other archaeologists and historians to be wary of taking the names for granted. Other archaeologists may not agree with the re-evaluation, but this is all part of the academic debate. And in the end, because debate identifies stresses and weaknesses in existing scholarship, it forms a necessary part of formulating better explanations.

Having said this, let us now turn to a step-by-step process for identifying the structure called an *abaton*.

The first question: "What does the name mean?" Before delving into the archaeological research, the archaeologist should begin by asking what the name *abaton* actually means. The ancient name might give a clue about how the building appeared. The term *abaton* literally means "untrodden" and might simply mean a sacred space.

The second question: "When and why?" Since the name provides few clues about the structure, the archaeologist should begin by asking when the building was originally identified and on what basis the interpretation was made. The site of Epidauros was excavated in the late nineteenth and early twentieth centuries, and there has yet to be a complete archaeological report made of it (Tomlinson 1983: 7). It would have been a difficult site to excavate. It had been used over the Greco-Roman period, and structures were added to the site while other structures had additions and changes made to them over time. The edifices found by the archaeologists would have been incomplete, with fallen walls and columns. Many were likely robbed for building materials. Therefore, determining the dating, phasing, and identification of buildings on a site of this scale is filled with complexities.

To make sense of the remains, the archaeologists turned to Pausanias to see if they could match the buildings they found with what he described. As we saw above, his descriptions are problematically vague. Moreover, he does not actually use the term *abaton* when he describes the sanctuary, though the term is found on inscriptions from the site. In any case, since the original archaeologists used Pausanias, we should consult his work. In doing so, we find that he does not make it clear how he travelled around the site. He explains that the sacred grove of Asclepius is surrounded on all sides by boundary markers (Paus. 2.27.1), but he does not tell us what is used to mark the area, nor does he provide an indication of its size. After describing the boundaries, he discusses the image of Asclepius, which was "half as big as the Olympian Zeus at Athens, and it was made of ivory and gold" (Paus. 2.27.2). He then refers to an inscription on the image which provides the name of artist – in this case, Thrasymedes, a Parian, son of Arignotus. Pausanias then describes the statue of the god as sitting and holding a staff in one hand, his other hand held above the head of a serpent, with a dog lying by the side of the statue (2.27.2). Pausanias' description does not actually state where this statue was placed, though it is likely that it was in the temple. Indeed, after the description of the statue, he writes, "over against the temple is where the suppliants slept" (2.27.2–3). Further confirmation that the statue of Asclepius was placed in the temple is found on a coin from Epidauros that dates to the Antonine period (*BMGC* 10.29). It depicts a large seated statue framed by a structure with a pediment, presumably the temple. However, earlier coins dating to the fourth century BC only depict the seated deity and do not show an edifice surrounding the image (Kraay 1966).

Returning to the comment "over against the temple is where the suppliants slept" (Paus. 2.27.2–3), it is noticeable that Pausanias does not use the word *abaton* but *entha* meaning "place". The building closest to the temple of Asclepius is a stoa (a long, rectangular structure, with a line of rooms along its back side, and a colonnaded porch running along its front side), which is the structure normally identified as the *abaton* in Epidauros and on many site plans of other Asclepia. However, Elderkin (1911) argued that the stoa was a hotel for visitors, while the *tholos* was the actual place where incubation occurred. He based his argument on the fact that this was the structure mentioned and described by Pausanias directly after he mentions "the place where the suppliants slept". Yet, Pausanias actually says, "Near has been built a circular building of white marble, called *Tholos* (round house), which is worth seeing" (2.27.3). He does not describe the function of the *Tholos*, he only speaks of the paintings he saw on the inside of it.

The third question: "Other sources?" Since the description Pausanias gave is imprecise, one should consider if there are any descriptions in other forms of literature that might help in its identification. As far as I could find in this preliminary study, no inscriptions that mention the word *abaton* have been found attached to a particular structure. Thus, they cannot be used to identify the building, only to note that something of that name was located at particular sites. At Epidauros, for example, the word *abaton* is mentioned on a few of the *iamata* in reference to incubation, but the word is used interchangeably with words for temple (*IG* IV², 1, no. 121. 6, 7, 11, 15, 17; *IG* IV², 1, no. 122. 24, 27, 29, 37, referenced in Edelstein and Edelstein 1998: 221–37). In comparison with the Asclepion in Athens, Aleshire (1989: 28–9, 28, no. 4) conducted a study of inscriptions from the site and argued that it is impossible to identify any of the structures positively. Aleshire (1989: 28–30) also stated that on the grounds of the literary evidence, the *abaton* could be a space within a temple rather than a separate structure itself. Aleshire's suggestion finds support in the interchangeable use of the term *iamata* and temple from Epidauros.

Moreover, the only surviving literary discussion that provides possible evidence for a visit to a sanctuary comes from Aristophanes, a Greek comic playwright. In his play *Ploutos* (*Wealth*), the implication is that the pilgrims were placed in the temple for incubation. A temple servant is described as putting out the lights, telling the pilgrims to sleep, and then removing the offerings from the altars. The temple servant and the fact that he takes votives from the altars are what suggest that the suppliants were placed in the temple. Aristophanes also mentioned an old woman sleeping near the male protagonist of the play, implying that people were not always separated on account of their sex (Ar. *Pl.* 668–83; 688–93). The literary evidence, therefore, does not give us a solid basis upon which we can (1) identify an *abaton* and (2) state that this was the one place where everyone received treatment in sanctuaries.

It is worthwhile seeing how the uncertainties of identification presented above can be overlooked by archaeologists. One of the latest catalogues on artefacts found at Asclepia by Reithmüller (2005) continues to use the original identifications of stoas as *abatons*. Reithmüller said that it was possible the "satellite sanctuaries" to Asclepius were based on plans from Epidauros. While he does note that the dimensions and architecture varied, he then becomes quite committed when saying that each site had an incubation hall, a fountain, a temple, and an altar. He states that the *abaton* could have been in a few places, such as a stoa, closed hall building, or peristyle complex (2005: 387). In theory, he may be correct, but the identification of the *abatons* that Reithmüller relies on is not guided by any concrete archaeological or literary information. Moreover, it must be remembered that the buildings he discusses are not only found in healing sanctuaries. Stoas, altars, and temples are common features in many Greco-Roman sanctuaries, such as Delphi and Olympia. Although Reithmüller concludes that there is not enough evidence to support his theory that all Asclepia are based on that at Epidauros, more information could have been provided about the archaeological evidence used to suggest places for the *abaton*.

The fourth question: "What is in the site report?" Since the literature provides few, if any, precise details about the *abaton*, the archaeologist will need to consult the site reports and examine what evidence was found in the buildings identified as *abatons*. Questions essential to making sense of the site report include asking how the structures in question were laid out and what artefacts were found in them. Since Epidauros is not properly published, this task is extremely difficult. So for the sake of simplicity, let us consider the Asclepion in Corinth (Lang 1977: figs. 13, 15; Figs. 15 and 16).

The sanctuary at Corinth was constructed on two levels, and the *temenos* was marked by a wall and a ramp, with a colonnade located on its northern side. On the upper level, just on the inside of the entrance, was a spring. The temple was the dominate structure on this level; it faced east, and its altar was located at the front of its entrance. It was built on top of an earlier temple, said to be for the god Apollo (Fig. 15). Two pits were dug next to it: one on the north side and the other on its south side. Behind the temple, foundations of a large structure were discovered. This was an open-plan building, and is believed to have been the *abaton*. From here, steps led to the lower section of the site (Fig. 16). Beneath the *"abaton"* were three rooms which were determined to be dining halls (letters A on the plan) because they had stands, possibly for couches, and each had a central hearth-like structure that showed signs of burning (Barefoot 2005: 210, fig. 12.4; Lang 1977: fig. 13). These rooms opened onto a large colonnade which had a water basin and springs (B and C on Fig. 16). None of the rooms can be positively identified. Some questions that therefore come to mind are whether the couches were beds for the ill to rest and whether the fires were intended to keep the occupants warm during cooler months of the year. In warmer weather, people could have kept cool in the shade of the peristyle courtyard and would have had access to water, all of which are important elements for maintaining a healthy balance of the humours. The layout of this site is interesting, but it is difficult for us to state with certainty whether the open-plan structure behind the temple was the *abaton*.

Could a stoa have been an *abaton*? Some archaeologists argue that this is plausible because stoas could have been used for sleeping. But this, too, is impossible to support because stoas are common to many sites. Furthermore, in accordance with other archaeological studies, stoas appear to have held a number of functions. It is plausible that people slept in them, but an archaeologist would need to check the artefacts in the rooms to see if they can provide a clue to the function(s) of the structure.

The fifth question: "What about the small finds?" With such limited information, the archaeologist should turn her attention to the artefacts found within the buildings. This is not as straightforward as it might seem because artefacts could have been thrown into a building after it had gone out of use. Or they might have been accidentally dropped. Or it may be that the finds represent only one function of the space (e.g. Allison 1997; 1999a: 5–8; 1999b; Hill 1995; Pollard 2001; Richards and Thomas 1984).

Looking at a structure that was identified as the Roman military hospital at Novae, in Moesia Superior (Dyczek 1995), one can see that the arrangement and type of finds revealed some interesting patterns. In fact, the small finds suggested that the structure did not serve a medical function. Many metal fragments – pieces of armour, a bronze helmet, phalerae, an iron spearhead, and

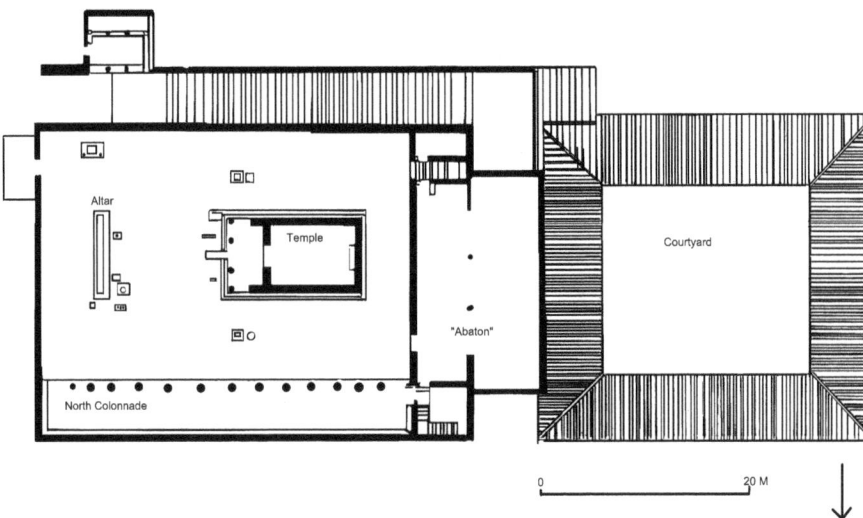

15. Upper section of the Asclepion at Corinth. After Lang (1977). Redrawn by the author.

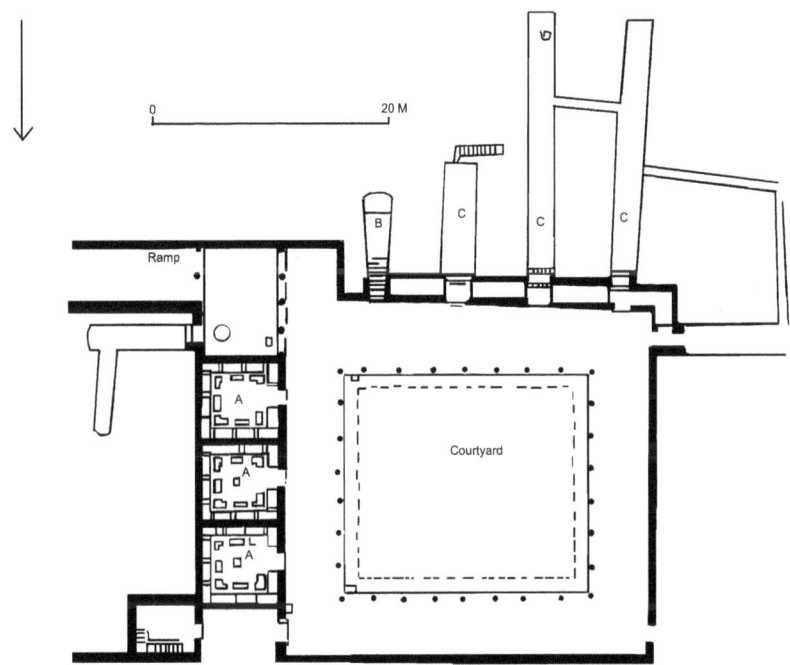

16. Lower section of the Asclepion at Corinth. After Lang (1977). Redrawn by the author. Letter A represents the possible dining rooms; letters B and C are cisterns.

fragments of chain – were found in the so-called bedrooms of the structure, along with lamps, vessel handles, and fibulae (Dyczek 1995: 200). Lamps, fibulae, and vessel handles are common domestic finds and appear in a number of structures, including barracks. The bits of armour could point to a place of storage, a barrack, or a workshop. The small vestibules between the "wards" had types of "tableware" and butchered animal bones (Dyczek 1995: 200–2), indicating a place for food preparation and/or dining. One could argue that the finds from this structure suggest a domestic space, perhaps a barrack. Room 48 of the building had broken probes and physicians' caskets (Dyczek 1995: 202). It can be suggested that treatments were offered to the soldiers in this particular room, rather than in the entire building. Yet, the tools could have served other purposes as well. The central courtyard of the structure had altars dedicated to Hygieia, Aesculapius, Jupiter, and Juno, suggesting that there might have been some form of sanctuary in the centre (Dyczek 1995: 202–3). There is no discussion on whether these finds were from the time of the building's use, abandonment, or destruction. Sometimes when buildings went out of use they were used to dump waste. What the small finds therefore reveal in this case is that structure was used for both medical and non-medical functions. In other words, it was not just a hospital; a variety of activities most likely occurred in this space.

In some instances, buildings have been identified on account of the small finds located within them, as seen with Neuss. When this is the case, two questions should immediately come to mind. First, were these the only medical tools found in the fortress and if not where were the others found? Second, what other objects were found with the tools in the so-called hospital?

In answer to the first question, eighty-four medical tools were found at the site and plotted on a distribution map. The pattern of deposition showed that other buildings had medical instruments in them. One can easily see the precariousness of the identification of the structure at Neuss. If all the other buildings had medical instrument deposits as well, then these too must be hospitals. Clearly, this conclusion is highly implausible. In response to the second question, it was found that the so-called hospital building, like the one at Novae, contained a variety of objects. This supposed *valetudinarium*, along with others, also showed signs of having served different functions, such as storage places or workshops (Johnson 1983: 185).

The sixth question: "What assumptions?" Archaeologists also need to reflect upon whether they are applying their own perceptions of how buildings should appear. Because we begin the identifications with what we know (see Parker Pearson and Richards 1994 and Thomas 1990: 15 for a discussion), we cannot escape relying on assumptions. But being aware that we use assumptions to make sense of things unfamiliar is a step that is frequently missed in archaeological research. Consider, for example, that although we do not have *abatons* today, we might be inclined to apply features of a modern hospital when conceptualizing this structure. One may therefore miss the fact that a hospital was only used to treat the ill until fairly recently. In the past, hospitals served a variety of purposes in both the Eastern and Western medical tradition: a place for the poor to be fed and for scholars to study (Baker 2012; Conrad 1995: 136; Horden 2008; Metzler 2012).

While these six questions will go a long way in acting as safeguards against hasty identification, there is no guarantee that mistakes will not be made. Like any discipline, archaeology often struggles with committing to making sense of its subject matter at the risk of ignoring anomalies that may indicate another meaning or theory.

6.3.4 Locating Spaces of Treatment Within Buildings

Having shown the difficulties involved in identifying a building in the ancient world, one might not be surprised to know that it can also be difficult to identify the function of a room within a building. Sometimes this task is easy if the architecture is clearly designed for a single purpose, such as the different types of rooms found in a Roman bath that were intended to be warm, hot, and cold. However, in most cases, rooms held multi-purpose functions. And if this is the case, the archaeologist's task becomes a very complex affair. What helps in these matters is a close contextual comparison of the artefacts found within a room or set of rooms.

If we look at Roman baths, we find the larger bathing complexes were usually found in cities throughout the Roman Empire. Some of these were quite substantial structures, which not only had the main bathing rooms but also contained latrines, swimming pools, palaestra, and rooms that might have been used as shops, meeting places, and/or libraries. It is also possible that some of these rooms might have been used for medical treatments.

A contextual examination of artefacts found in a bath was made by Künzl (1986, 1989/90), who argued to have found a room that was used for surgery in the baths at Trier. Künzl based his conclusion on the few instruments found in the room and how the room's arrangement was similar to those in what he thought were military hospitals. However, G. Fagan (1999: 90–3) disagreed with Künzl contending that his interpretation was overdetermined. G. Fagan notes that the instruments are few in number and the layout of the rooms is linear, unlike the layout found in the so-called *valetudinaria*. It is likely that doctors could have worked the Roman baths, especially since people might have been visiting the baths for cures for illness (e.g. G. Fagan 1999: 91–3; Jackson 1990a: 11, 1990b: 9, 1993: 88; Künzl 1986, 1989/90; Yegül 1992: 335). There is further evidence of medical treatments in baths from the Roman legionary fortress at Caerleon, Wales. Teeth were discovered in the drains of the baths with possible dental implement marks on them

(Zienkiewicz 1986: 223). Although there is support for Künzl's general argument that medical activity occurred in the baths, G. Fagan's counter-argument makes it evident that it is actually difficult to identify a precise place for this activity. As suggested by the medical writers we encountered above, it is possible that people moved their beds to spaces that were conducive to the treatment they required, rather than being confined to a particular room in a building. Thus, when attempting to identify a space within a structure, it is advisable to describe *all* of the artefacts found within the room and to note the room's plan. It is also important to see if similar structures had artefacts of the same type located in the same places.

6.4 IDENTIFYING ATTITUDES TOWARDS MEDICINE AND HYGIENE IN SPACES

Identifying spaces and structures is only half of what archaeologists do when examining the remains of structures, landscapes, and public amenities. These remains can also be examined to access social rules, behaviours, and conceptions about health (e.g. the body, hygiene, and medical treatments) not described in literature. If there is some reference to conceptions of space in ancient texts, the archaeological record can be checked to see if the remains corroborate what the ancient writer said.

When I explain theoretical approaches concerned with aspects of space and archaeology to my students, I begin by asking them two questions. First, how do they react when they come into contact with sick people? And second, how do they behave when they are visiting a patient or being treated in a hospital? They usually respond that they physically distance themselves from the ill person because they do not want to "catch their germs". As for the buildings, they often say they do not like hospitals or sick rooms, finding them depressing, scary, and a possible source of infection. They also acknowledge that they will avoid touching objects and speak in quiet tones when they are in a hospital. Everything they mention involves a spatial element that is dictated by their perception of how diseases are spread, even if the condition is not contagious.

Because archaeologists are no exception to normative conceptions, they have to be aware of the way in which modern conceptions of space may be at work when attempting to imagine past locations. Studies by the anthropologists Rapoport and Bourdieu have demonstrated how archaeologists think about and interpret building spaces. Rapoport (1969) was one of the first to bring to our attention the fact that modern Western notions of space influence scholarly interpretations of structures. He pointed out that our conceptions of hygiene, smells, lighting, and comfort might not have been the same as the people we are studying. We often assume these would have been the case because it is what we know.

So one of the strategies for guarding against the importation of modern notions is deliberate consideration of those categories which are substantively defined by any person's social context. Thus, for archaeologists, considerations of spatial conceptions usually begin with questions of how to interpret spatial patterns in view of class, gender, death, and ritual/religious experience (Bender 1993; Gilchrist 1994; Grøn, Engelstad, and Lindblom 1991; Johnson 2000: 111–13; Moore 1996; Parker Pearson and Richards 1994; Rapoport 1969). For example, in his study of the Kabyle house, Bourdieu (1973, 1977) found that the Kabyle understandings of gender were represented in how they laid out their houses, as there were clearly defined places that were intended for the activities performed by females and males. His analysis demonstrates that societies will have different reasons for building and organizing their structures and spaces. Beyond architectural divisions, Bourdieu also concerned himself with the body's incorporation within spatial layouts, arguing these layouts were a source fundamental to the maintenance of social rules. Furthermore, he used the term *habitus* to denote how bodily actions and behaviour, rather than through spoken words, express and reinforce these rules (often unawaringly). Bourdieu's point is quite interesting, since it prioritizes non-verbal activity as a means of understanding. Through the observation of movements, expressions, body language, spatial placement, and so on, a person learns appropriate ways to act in specific circumstances – much like my students moving away from someone who is ill (Bender 1998: 35; Bourdieu 1977: 89; Strathern 1999: 26).

In a similar vein, anthropologists have found that rules concerning space are culturally constructed. Associated with built space, one often finds rules regarding correct bodily distance between people. In the 1960s, the study of proxemics became a popular method to determine how people reacted to their environmental surroundings and to other people in accordance with their cultural norms and perceptions of space (Argyle 1988: 184; Deetz 1977: 25). For example, it was established that, in certain cultures, people stand closer to one another in conversation than in other cultures (Argyle 1988: 58). These social rules not only affect the manner in which people use non-verbal communication with their body, but also the way they organize structures in which conversation occurs (Argyle 1988: 185–7; Rapoport 1990: 10). The difficulty with the original study of proxemics is that it developed as a positivistic science devoted to measuring actual distances. It has therefore been criticized for a form of analysis that removes human decision making and socially specific values from its "equation". Nonetheless, the value in this study is the realization that there are cultural rules involved in people's reactions to the spaces surrounding them.

The archaeology of spatial studies, particularly landscape studies, has also been influenced by the phenomenological treatises of Merleau-Ponty (1962) and Heidegger (1978). While phenomenological theory is quite complex, the works of Merleau-Ponty and Heidegger are used to show how primary to our way of understanding is our mode of being-in the surrounding environment. From an archaeological perspective, it has helped us to think of what spaces might have meant to people in the past, and what people would have experienced when they encountered different environments. In turn, it has enabled archaeologists to see the complex relation between humans and their environments in terms of how, on the one hand, the environments might have been shaped by their cultural perceptions and, on the other hand, how the surroundings might have reinforced or created people's expected social rules of behaviour. What people sense – see, hear, smell, feel – when they encounter a space are determined by their social norms, and recognizing this can help to explain why spaces were constructed in certain manners and what the spaces meant to the individual or group of people who used or, to quote Heidegger, "dwelled" in them.

For example, when visiting the healing sanctuary at Epidauros, the pilgrims did not see the temple as soon as they entered. They had to cleanse themselves ritually, walk through the sacred space, and only then would they see the inscriptions as they travelled to the temple of Asclepius. All of these activities would inform their behaviour, and perhaps create a sense of expectation as they approached the temple (see Grøn 1991: 7–8 for a discussion). Such observations can also be found in cultural taboos or fears related to the body. The fear of leprosy in medieval Europe, for instance, manifests in the built environment in terms of where leper hospitals were placed – that is, outside or on the edge of the city boundaries (Metzler 2012; Turner 1984: 68–9).

What, then, might the placement and layout of public amenities, and ancient conceptions of landscapes tell us about health in the past? Below we will examine a few types of structures – water supply, baths, latrines – all of which are interesting structures for the study of ancient technologies. We will also consider landscapes to see how the above-mentioned archaeological theories help us determine medical conceptions from surviving remains.

6.4.1 Water Supply

A clean water supply is mentioned in numerous ancient literary texts as being essential for health and a healthy environment (e.g. Frontin., *Aq*). This idea finds support in the archaeological remains of aqueducts, fountains, wells, and cisterns. Their importance, particularly the aqueducts, is not only attested through the network of systems that brought water into cities, but in the quality of their construction, their size, and by the commemorative inscriptions found on some of them.

Since a number of ancient writers mention water supply, a good first study for archaeologists is to see if what they describe can be found in the archaeological record. In larger urban areas, water tended to be carried into cities by aqueducts, such as those seen in Rome (Aicher 1995; Hodge 1992). When the water arrived at its destination, settling tanks were placed at the end of the aqueducts to allow for impurities to be removed from the water before it was dispensed to three areas: fountains, baths, and private houses (Vitruvius, *De Arch.* 8.6.1–2). This practice has been identified at Pompeii. For those living in houses without a private supply of water, the water was usually collected from fountains that were attached to the system (Laurence 2007: 48).

Although the descriptions and the archaeology verify each other, the remains of fountains can be used to see how far people might have travelled to collect their water. In the case of Pompeii, the location of fountains has been used to try and determine neighborhood areas (Laurence 2007: 45–52). The fountains are located on every street, usually near a crossroads, meaning that people did not have to travel far to collect their daily supply of water and could possibly have made several trips if it was necessary. The ready availability of "fresh" water is a demonstration of the importance placed on this particular aspect of health in the ancient world.

The collection of water was also an activity that has been described as gender or class specific. It was either women and/or slaves who had the job of collecting it, attested by the numerous Greek pottery paintings depicting women at fountains (e.g. Williams 1983). On a deeper interpretative level, even if it is only perceived of as minor, the spatial relationship between the activities performed by a specific group of people and a public amenity were an important way of ensuring the maintenance of a particular aspect of a healthy regimen in a household.

On a wider geographical scale, archaeologists could also make comparisons of the location of public and private water supplies between other urban and rural areas, fortifications, and households in order to see if there existed regional differences about what constituted a healthy water supply. For example, although there is no doubt that the location of wells was based on access to water, their location can also be examined to see if they were placed in areas seen to be salubrious. We would expect an area perceived as dirty or unhygienic not to have been used for the placement of a water supply for drinking. Yet, once again, the archaeology has revealed some surprising results.

The site of 1 Poultry in Roman London consisted of an area with houses that had wells in their yards. Domestic rubbish, along with evidence of pigs and chickens, were found by the wells. The dwellings were also located close to tanneries and forges, and the run-off from these places – which could include urine, faecal matter, and metals – could have contaminated the water supply (Perring and Brigham 2000: 412–14; Redfern 2003: 153–4; Rowsome 2000: 34–5). Hence, the comparison here indicates possible differences in perceptions of a fresh and healthy water supply.

6.4.2 Concepts of Hygiene in the Baths and Latrines

In relation to what was just observed with the water supply in London, it should then be asked what the archaeology of other structures might reveal about concepts of hygiene. In literature, bathing was an important part of daily regimen and was prescribed for a number of medical treatments (Celsus, *Med.* 3.22; Galen, *De Sanitate Tuenda*). Baths have again been found in the Greek and Roman archaeological record, but, like the structures associated with water supply, there is more evidence for these having existed in the Roman world than the Greek. For Greece, there are references to bathing establishments and vapour baths (e.g. Panayotatou 1919: 111–12). Many of them seem to have been small household baths or, in the case of public establishments, rooms with heated cauldrons of water. It seems as if people poured the water from the cauldrons over themselves.

Roman baths are easy to identify, but they are not uniform in design and vary in layout and size across the Empire. As a rule, Roman baths usually contained a hypocaust system, water supply, drainage, and sometimes latrines. The hypocaust system consisted of two rooms: the *caldarium* (hot room) and *tepidarium* (warm room). They had raised floors to facilitate underfloor heating, and flue tiles that conveyed heat up the walls. The *frigidarium* (cold room) was the room just after the hypocaust system, farthest from the furnace. It often had a cold plunge bath.

Just to provide a contrast to modern sentiments and expectations, while we would expect bathing to have been a hygienic activity in the ancient world, the establishments were often warm and moist, and with a number of visitors each day, the environment was an ideal catalyst for the spread of pathogens and communicable diseases. Moreover, the waters were apparently not always clean and sometimes mixed with mud. It is also uncertain how often the bath water was changed. With the use of bathing oils, the surface of the bath water, as well as on the walls and floors, would have been coated with oil from people's bodies. The fumes and smoke from the furnace might have also been problematic. Finally, we do not know if people may have urinated in the bathing water (G. Fagan 1999: 176–88).

Latrines are also argued to be signs of hygienically conscious Romans. Many public facilities were located in baths, urban areas, and even Roman forts. The one found in the south-east corner of Housesteads Roman Fort on Hadrian's Wall is an excellent surviving example (Rushworth 2009: 222). The latrine at Housesteads was constructed next to the fortress wall, and the toilet seats were placed above a channel of running water that flushed the waste outside the fort. Although the seats do not survive, they were likely to have been keyhole style seats such as those found in other areas of Rome, such as at Ostia (Jackson 1988: 50, fig. 9). Located in front of the seats was a small water channel, which is thought to have been for washing hands, holding the sponges that were likely used in lieu of toilet paper, or perhaps both. A common item used for toilet cleansing seems to have been a sponge on a stick (Martial, *Ep.* 12.48), which, if reused, could harbour bacteria and, if it was shared, a possible source of contagion.

Water from the baths was sometimes used to flush sewers and latrines, which helped to remove waste, foul smells, and alleviate the spread of pathogens. However, the sewage tended not to be flushed far beyond city or fortress boundaries, which would mean that fetid air was a problem, not to mention the growth of bacteria that would have contributed to the spread of disease.

Few houses had toilets; it seems that most people had either chamber pots that were emptied onto streets, or seats constructed over cesspits that were found to have been placed next to the kitchen in Pompeian houses (Jackson 1988: 51).

Hence, the archaeology reveals that living conditions, even in areas thought to have been built for hygienic purposes, do not equate with modern conceptions of cleanliness. Nonetheless, they provide a surprising insight into conceptions of hygiene in the ancient world that, if looked at more carefully and compared between different areas, can reveal localized practices and understandings of what constituted a clean and healthy environment in the past.

6.4.3 Views of the Body Found in Baths and Latrines

While baths were recommended for health and played a role in people's daily regimen, the actual construction of baths and latrines also provide us with ideas about people's views of privacy and personal modesty. These norms, like today, can provide an account of how patients may have reacted towards medical treatments. For example, in modern hospitals and doctor's surgeries, patients are usually provided with gowns and treated in private rooms because of conceptions of modesty. In many cases, these are not actually necessary for treatment, but the objects and spaces tell us that the patient's concerns with modesty are also socially dictated.

Small finds indicate that children, women, and men had access to the baths. However, it is often thought that Roman men and women bathed in separate spaces or, in the case of small baths, at separate times. These views are based on some insubstantial evidence mentioned in ancient literature about emperors dividing public baths between the sexes (e.g. *S.H.A., Hadr.*, 18.10), and some larger bathing structures having two sets of baths, which were thought to be spaces for men and women. Along with this, it is generally believed that bathing was performed naked, which may be offensive to some modern historians and archaeologists. Citing lack of conclusive evidence, G. Fagan notes that we do not know if people bathed naked. However, he does say that there is some archaeological information that does suggest naked bathing occurred. He refers to a mosaic located at Piazza Armerina, Sicily, which depicts a naked man with oil and a *strigil* (G. Fagan 1999: fig. 30).

Since there are differences in building layout and different indigenous populations within the Roman Empire, it is highly possible that localized attitudes towards the body, gender differences, and culturally determined behaviours influenced the rules about bathing (Bowen Ward 1992). It would be useful for archaeologists to compare baths from different areas to see if there are noticeable regional differences in design.

Public latrines also point to toilet etiquette that can be quite shocking by modern Western standards. The seats were placed very close together, indicating that there was no privacy. From what can be determined, it seems as if women and men also shared the facilities (Jansen 1997; Koloski-Ostrow 1996; Neudecker 1994). One can perhaps conclude from this that the layout of the baths and latrines indicates Romans did view their bodies rather freely in some respects. In relation to medicine, we often assume that treatments were done privately, but if people were comfortable showing their bodies in certain spaces and performing certain bodily functions in public, it is possible that they were also unafraid of having medical treatments performed on them in public spaces. This could explain the lack of easily identifiable medical facilities.

6.4.4 Salubrious Environments

Having mentioned structures that were constructed in accordance with health, one also needs to think about the Greco-Roman relationship to the surrounding environment and landscape. As there has been quite a bit of study on landscape and space in archaeology (for an overview, see e.g., Ashmore and Knapp 1999; Blake 2007; Johnson 2007; Preucel and Meskell 2007), there is quite a diverse body of theory that can help archaeologists rethink ancient practices. Sometimes archaeologists designate the activities local to an area as "taskscapes". This term was coined by Ingold, and it refers to the immutable boundaries between the landscape and activities (e.g. Gamble 2008; Ingold 1993). To this, one could add the term "healthscapes", which would focus attention on archaeological studies that consider how salubrious environments might have been conceived and constructed in the past.

Archaeologists will examine a space to determine how people might have moved through the landscape in an attempt to ascertain what they might have experienced (Barrett 1993; Johnson 2007: 134–62; Thomas 1991; Tilley 1994). Ultimately, this phenomenological approach allows us to re-create people's sense of being within a particular place and time. In relation to health, it would also be necessary to consider how someone with an illness or difficulties in movement had to negotiate the space and structures.

There are a few ways archaeologists will try to access past experiences in landscapes. The more technical means of doing this is to generate a computer simulation through the use of geographic information systems (GIS). This technology is not simply used to collect spatial data, since the information can be analysed to reconstruct the appearance of landscapes in the past (Gaffney and Gater 2003; Gaffney, Stancic, and Watson 1995: 213; Gillings 2005). In addition to giving archaeologists a sense of what a past location was like, GIS data also allow them to run their landscape simulations through different lights, seasons, and weather conditions.

A simpler way to determine how people might have perceived their surroundings is visualization. Here, an archaeologist will walk through an area in an attempt to re-create the landscape experience. For example, if we were to try this in a healing sanctuary with the aim of determining a pilgrim's experience, we would need to consider a few issues. (1) The site will not be in the same condition as it was in the past. The archaeologist would have to decide which period they were interested in studying, and then imagine only the structures that were standing at that particular time. (2) We would also have to imagine being ill or having impairments that made movement difficult.

(3) Landscapes might have had more trees or fields in the past, so this would need to be considered (Chapter 7; see also Goldberg 1999; Kent 1990: 3).

Concepts of salubrious environments can also be determined through the ancient literature. For example, Vegetius (*de Mil.* 6.1) said that Roman fortifications should be placed in areas that had clean water that were not marshy. Areas that were too sunny and hot needed shade, and those that were in cold regions should have ample sunlight and be protected from the wind. This is supported by a statement of Vitruvius (*De Arch.* 6.1) who says that the human body requires a certain climate to live comfortably and that buildings and rooms should be constructed in a manner to assure this comfort. He argued that rooms ideally should be arranged according to the season in which they were being used. The summer dining room in a villa should face north because it will be cool and dry. Or there is the example of Plutarch who asked in the *Roman Questions* in his *Moralia* (286 D):

> why is the shrine of Aesclapius (in Rome) outside the city?
>
> Is it because they considered it more healthful to spend their time outside the city than within the city walls? In fact, the Greeks as might be expected have their shrines of Aesclapius situated in places which are clean and high.
>
> Or is it because they believe that god came at their summons from Epidauros and the Epidaurians have their shrine of Aesclapius at some distance from the city.
>
> Or is it because the serpent came out from the trireme into the island, and there disappeared and thus they thought that the god himself was indicating to the site for building.

Two of the possibilities mentioned above suggest a Roman understanding of what constituted a healthy environment – namely, that was in a place that was high and clean and that it was outside the city walls. The text from Plutarch could be compared to known healing sites to see if his assertions were accurate. In actual fact, sanctuaries to Asclepius and other healing deities are found in both rural and urban areas. Yet despite this discrepancy between site and literary source, a comparison of sites would enable a more detailed study of landscape features and/or orientations.

6.5 CONCLUSION

This chapter has explored the ways in which archaeologists employ a variety of methods to help better understand where places for treating illness may have existed in the ancient world and how conceptions of illness and healing affected the manner in which landscapes and structures were understood and constructed. Because the identification of structures that may have been used for healing is by no means easy, we have also seen how archaeologists can safeguard against interpretive oversights. In short, employing comparative analysis of sites and small finds and bearing in mind cultural biases can help to present a clearer representation of the past. Taken together, the artefact patterns and structural positions in the landscapes can provide a robust and even surprising view of space and how an ancient society saw others, themselves, and the practices that bound them together in view of being healthy.

CONSIDERATION QUESTIONS

1. Consider your reactions to spaces of medicine. How do you behave in a hospital, doctor's surgery, or a spa? Is your behaviour dictated by the construction of the space? Is the spatial layout dictated by expected behaviours, activities, and conceptions of health and hygiene? Then consider what is written in ancient texts about spaces.
2. How do you react to an individual who is ill? Do you adapt yourself and surrounding spaces to suit yours or their needs? Do you think people might have had similar or different reactions in the past? Do you think a spatial awareness of the ill affects the construction of spaces?

FURTHER READING

Baker, P. 2012. "Medieval Islamic Hospitals: Structural Design and Social Concepts". In *Medicine and Space: Body, Surroundings and Borders in Antiquity and the Middle Ages*, P. Baker, H. Nijdam, and C. van't Land, eds. Proceedings of the Anglo-Dutch Wellcome Symposium, Nijmegen, November 2007. Leiden: Brill, pp. 245–72.

Baker, P., H. Nijdam, C. van 't Land, and eds. 2012. *Medicine and Space: Body, Surroundings and Borders in Antiquity and the Middle Ages*. Leiden: Brill.

Grøn, O. 1991. "Introduction". In *Social Space: Human Spatial Behaviour in Dwellings and Settlements*, O. Grøn, E. Engelstad, and I. Lindblom, eds. Odense: Odense University Press, pp. 7–8.

Kent, S. 1990. "Activity Areas and Architecture: An Interdisciplinary View of the Relationship between Use of Space and Domestic Built Environment". In *Domestic Architecture and the Use of Space: An Interdisciplinary Cross-Cultural Study*, S. Kent, ed. Cambridge: Cambridge University Press, pp. 1–8.

Parker Pearson, M., and C. Richards 1994. "Ordering the World: Perceptions of Architecture, Space and Time". In *Architecture and Order: Approaches to Social Space*. London: Routledge, pp. 1–37.

CHAPTER 7

ARCHAEOLOGICAL SCIENCE

7.1 INTRODUCTION

Archaeological science is the subject of this final chapter. The topics covered are biological anthropology and paleopathology; aDNA (ancient Deoxyribonucleic Acid) and stable isotope analysis; environmental archaeology; residue samples; and metal wear analysis. We will begin with studies of bodily remains. These can be examined for congenital conditions, trauma, and diseases suffered by an individual or group of people. Environmental analyses help in the evaluation of ancient diets, weather conditions, and pathogens that might have affected people's living conditions and health. More recent forensic developments help archaeologists find trace elements of blood on cutting tools and possible medicinal ingredients in pottery containers. Studies of aDNA and stable isotopes found in human remains help to sex bodies biologically, and to detect congenital conditions, diets, and migration patterns. Skeletal and environmental remains can be classified as forms of material cultural to answer the types of questions described in the previous chapters, but other information available from them has great potential for enhancing our awareness of disease, health, and medical treatments in the past.

As exciting as these prospects are, it must be stated that the information presented below is not without disputation over the accuracy of certain scientific techniques used in analysing material remains. These fields also change rapidly, which means that some methods can quickly become obsolete. So generally, it is worth being cautious about information that underwent some form of lab-based analysis significantly prior to one's own immediate time period. It is always best to consult with an expert and to read the most recent publications on different aspects of science-based archaeology, if possible.

Many archaeologists, myself included, do not have training in these aspects of the field. So skeletal, environmental, and any form of scientific analysis of material remains must be examined by people who specialize in biological/physical anthropology, archaeobotany, environmental archaeology, or paleoentymology, or who have lab-based training for other forms of material studies. In some cases, such as with studies of aDNA and isotopes, the analyses are made by chemists. These studies also require special laboratory equipment and laboratories for examination, meaning that some of the processes can be expensive. It would be counterproductive to present a full-scale introduction to archaeological science, given the intricacies of this type of work and the general purpose of this book. Rather, the intention of this chapter is to make the reader aware of the types of information that can be ascertained from the above-mentioned archaeological studies and explain how they can be used in medical history.

This chapter begins with an explanation of scientific archaeology to provide the reader with an awareness of how this archaeological discipline relates to the studies of material remains described in the previous chapters. Following on from this, descriptions of the types of analyses available to archaeologists will be given. This section will begin with ancient bodies, and includes discussions on aDNA and stable isotope examinations. Environmental archaeology is the next topic covered. In this section, explanations of how past landscapes, weather conditions, and flora and fauna are studied are presented. The third and final section of the chapter concludes with information about forensic studies that can be made to identify trace residues of ingredients in pottery, use-wear on sharp objects, and even the remains of blood on tools, all of which might provide us with information about medical practices in the classical world.

7.2 THE SCIENTIFIC DIVISION IN ARCHAEOLOGY

Since the fields of archaeology discussed in this chapter are grounded in different research methods from those mentioned in the previous chapters, divisions in the subject have developed. These boundaries are evident through the existence of separate scholarly journals dedicated to scientific areas of archaeology, such as the *American Journal of Osteology*, *Archaeofauna*, and the *Journal of Archaeological Science*. Some studies even appear in science journals, which may be completely overlooked by archaeologists. Conferences orientated towards these areas are held annually, and tend to be attended by specialists alone. There are even archaeology and anthropology departments that focus on scientific archaeology or material archaeology. On the one hand, these separate journals, conferences, and departments are impeding cross-disciplinary activities. However, on the other, these subjects are rarely included in "mainstream" archaeological publications and conferences, so there is a need for these events and publications. Nonetheless, the division stems from both sections of archaeology.

Because of this division, this means that a number of fascinating studies on human or environmental remains from the Greco-Roman period, for example, might be overlooked in more conventional examinations made by material specialists. Conversely, scientific archaeologists may also miss information from material studies. Consequently, medical historians, who may look at material archaeology, may never know of the existence of some of these studies that could have a direct bearing on their work.

Archaeologists are mindful that this division is problematic and limiting, and many scholars have called for greater cross-disciplinary research and discussion (e.g. Roberts 2002: 15–16; Roberts and Cox 2003: 383–5; Sofaer 2006: 5–10). Besides simply working together, it is also important for interaction to occur because it may be difficult for someone unfamiliar with the scientific methodologies to judge whether a case study is based on critical scholarship – including an awareness of which laboratories are better equipped to undertake archaeological studies. A general appreciation of the possibilities of these areas of archaeology can help in expanding interdisciplinary research, and can contribute greatly to the field of ancient medicine.

7.3 BODILY REMAINS

In this section, the types of examinations that can be made on ancient bodies, consisting of skeletal, cremated, and mummified remains, will be described. Those who study human and animal remains are known as biological or physical anthropologists, and a subfield to this discipline is the study of paleopathology, which specifically focuses on the identification of diseases (Renfrew and Bahn 2008: 447; Roberts and Cox 2003: 13). When examining the remains, they will try to determine the biological sex, age, overall stature, and possible conditions of the individual being studied, aspects which are detailed below. Bones and soft tissue, if it survives, can reveal evidence for certain congenital conditions, diseases, and traumas, and in some instances, evidence for surgical treatment.

Animal bones are also identified and studied by biological anthropologists and are useful for identifying regional fauna for environmental purposes, or to determine animals kept for livestock, giving us an idea of the past environment and diets of people in particular regions. Although the focus of this section is on human remains, it is important to remind the reader that similar examinations can be made on animal bones, which may be important for studies of ancient veterinary science.

Human remains are found in a number of locations. Complete or nearly complete skeletons are contained within inhumation burials, which tend to be grouped together in necropoleis. Sometimes they are found as single burials in isolated locations, or in places where an individual might have died without receiving a proper burial. This latter type of human remain is quite rare because without receiving a proper burial, the corpse would likely have been preyed upon by wild animals, meaning the bones could have been disarticulated and left on the surface of the ground. Even if disarticulated bones are found, and depending on their condition, they can still be examined for evidence of disease, stature, and trauma. Ideally, a complete articulated skeleton is best for examinations because it allows the physical anthropologist to gain a holistic view of a person's health.

Cremated remains are usually found buried in urns in necropoleis. Bones that have undergone cremation tend to survive better than non-cremated bones in the archaeological record because the firing process gives the bones greater strength, and it destroys the organic component of bones that are attractive to micro-organisms (Mays 1998: 209; McKinley and Bond 2005). Age and biological sex can be determined if correct portions of the bones survive. In certain instances, aDNA can be taken from cremated bones if the collagen has not been oxidized.

Mummified remains provide the archaeologist with more information about life in the past because the soft tissues of the body survive. However, they only tend to be found in dry climates, such as Egypt and the Andes. Bodies found preserved in peat bogs and in cold arctic climates are also well preserved, but these are only found in limited areas. Remains of this type are studied by a team of people that generally consists of Egyptologists (in the case of mummies), biological/physical anthropologists, and a medical pathologist (for autopsies). The Egyptologist will attempt to reconstruct the social conditions of the period in which the individual lived, whilst the physical anthropologists and medical pathologist will work together in determining the condition of the body.

Both non-invasive and invasive techniques are used to determine the health of the mummified individual. Non-invasive procedures involve taking photographs of the individual to make detailed records of their condition and any notable marks located on their body. Infrared cameras can be used to detect tattoos that might have disappeared over time. Although not from the period in question, the Ice Man, found frozen in a melting Alpine glacier on the Italian and Austrian border, had tattoos on his body that were thought to be associated with arthritis (Renfrew and Bahn 2008: 69).

X-rays and computerized axial tomography (CAT) scans are also used to peer inside the body. A study of mummified remains from Hellenistic and Roman Egypt belonging to the British Museum was able to demonstrate that sex and age range could be determined through CAT scans (Filer 1997, 1998, 1999, 2002). Magnetic resonance imaging (MRI) works by lining the body's hydrogen atoms in a magnetic field, making them emit radio waves. This method is only useful in bodies that contain water (Renfrew and Bahn 2008: 448–9). The use of a fibre-optic endoscope, a flexible tube with a tiny light and camera, can also be used to examine the interior of bodies to see which of the organs exist and to determine their condition (Renfrew and Bahn 2008: 449). Sometimes samples of the skin will be taken and rehydrated for use in microscopic examination. It is also likely that aDNA analysis can be undertaken on these remains (e.g. Cockburn, Cockburn, and Reyman 1998; Zimmerman 2005).

As mummified bodies are rare outside of Egypt for the period in question, articulated skeletal remains are the most useful in examinations of Greco-Roman health care.

7.3.1 Biological Sex

Biological sex, as briefly mentioned in Chapter 5, is different from gender. To reiterate, biological sex is determined by the physical traits that define whether a person is male, female, or hermaphrodite. Gender, on the other hand, is the social role that makes someone male, female, or other in their particular society. Gender identities are fluid and may depend on age, social situation, and biological determinates such as genitalia. In some cases, a person can be physically one sex but will take on a role that is traditional for the opposite sex in their society. Hence, biological sex is not always indicative of the roles people had when they were alive. Nonetheless, biological sex is important to determine for human remains because certain diseases or conditions of the body might be specific to one sex, such as pregnancy in women. Moreover, sex can be used in studies to determine if certain groups of people were more susceptible to illness than others, for example.

To ascertain the sex of a skeleton, it is best to examine the entire body. It is also almost impossible to determine the sex of a subadult. This is because children do not have high testosterone levels, the hormone responsible for the development of male characteristics, so they will not have the same biological markers that are used to determine sex in adult skeletons. The diamorphic differences between males and females are as follows. Generally, male adult skeletons tend to be more robust than females. However, more precise indications of sex are found in the pelvic bones. A male's pelvis tends to be narrower, while a female's is wider and more suited for pregnancy and childbirth. The angle of the female's pubic bone, located at the front of the pelvis, is also wider than a male's. Like the complete skeleton, the male skull is usually more robust than the female's, and it often has a brow ridge, whereas the female's tends to be smaller and without a ridge over the brow (Mays 1998: 33–8). Teeth, too, are sometimes used to determine biological sex. There is a difference in the thickness of tooth enamel between males and females. The X chromosome promotes the growth of enamel and dentine, whereas the Y chromosome only helps in the growth of enamel. In some cases, males will have larger teeth than the local female population (Becker 2002; Cox 2005: 238–9). However, all of these biological determinates can also be influenced by diet, exercise, and genetics, so they are not completely foolproof. In some cases, adult skeletons show little sexual dimorphism. In these instances, the report will note that the sex is indeterminate (Mays 1998: 33–8).

DNA analysis can also be employed as a method of sex determination, especially with infants, juveniles, incomplete skeletons, and those remains that have low dimorphic levels. Nonetheless, ancient DNA does not always survive and studies of it are about eighty per cent reliable at the moment (Cox 2005: 239). These examinations are also costly, so the traditional methods of establishing sex just described are still commonly employed by biological anthropologists.

7.3.2 Age

Like biological sex, it is useful to know the age of an individual to establish whether certain groups of people were more susceptible to particular diseases and environmental conditions than others. Age is generally measured by the growth and fusion of certain bones and the eruption of teeth. Precise ages cannot be applied to skeletal remains because people develop at different rates. For example, some children reach puberty at the age of twelve and others at thirteen or fourteen years of age. Biological anthropologists, therefore, classify people into certain age groups according to the development of their teeth and bones. The classifications are: *neonates; infants*, usually those under three years of age; *children*, roughly three to seven years of age; *juveniles*, eight to ten years of age; *adolescents*, ten to twenty years old; and *adults* who are twenty years or older (Scheuer and Black 2000). Depending on the condition of the teeth, it is sometimes possible to establish the age of an adult more precisely. The deterioration and loss of some teeth occur at specific phases in a person's life. Yet, dental condition can be affected by diet, dental hygiene, and activity, such as using teeth in non-masticatory functions, which make it difficult to use this method with much certainty (Larsen 1997: 258–62).

Age in skeletons can also give us an indication of an individual's social status. It has been found that there are often correlations between age and burial location in the Greco-Roman world. Infants, children, and adults tend to be buried in different manners and areas of necropoleis from one another (e.g. Houby-Nielsen 2000; Meskell 1994; Scott 1991). In rare instances, adults are sometimes found buried with children or in the same manner as children, which might be indicative of their status. Comparing the bodily condition with the manner and place of burial can give us an insight into a person's perceived age and social status. For example, an out-of-use well in the Athenian Agora, dating to the late Hellenistic period, contained the remains of 450 infants, one adult male, and one juvenile (Little 1999; Papadopoulos 2000). The adult had signs of severe arthritis, which may have been crippling (Little 1999). If this were the case, when alive, his condition may have left him requiring care and assistance to ensure his survival. It is possible that the help offered to him was considered by people in his society to be similar to that offered to a child or infant. Hence, although he was an adult, by modern senses, in body and age, his condition might have given him a child-like status. This example, along with many others, serves to warn us that even though we might be able to identify a person's biological age group, this information may not provide an accurate reflection of his or her social status or mental or physical condition, just as we saw in the relationship between someone's biological sex and gender identity.

7.3.3 Stature and General Health

Once the sex and age are established, human remains can be examined to ascertain the general health of the individual, and in cases where there are larger samples of skeletal material, the local population can be considered. Although someone's stature can be related to biological sex, it is also influenced by their genetic structure, general health, diet, and exercise. The long bones of the body are examined initially by physical anthropologists to ascertain a person's height and weight, which may have been associated with their health. Comparisons to other skeletal remains from the same region can be a useful indicator of the overall stature of the population, which may be based on the general environmental factors of the area. A society with good sanitation, an overall healthy diet, and fewer disease outbreaks tend to have a taller population than societies where these are lacking (Weiss 2009: 38–40).

Since some people can have a small stature on account of their genes, the signs of arrested development are more reliable determinates of health in the past. How do these signs manifest themselves on the skeleton? When trying to determine the overall health of an individual, the biological anthropologist will examine the remains for signs known as "general stress indicators". The development of the skeleton and teeth are affected by an individual's health, which might have led to diminished growth or susceptibility to certain diseases and bodily conditions. The general indicators of health tend to be bodily stature, vertebral canal size, the condition of tooth enamel, and Harris lines (small lines found on bones).

The vertebral canal is completely formed by age four. A small canal is indicative of an individual having suffered a disease and/or malnutrition prior to their fourth birthday (Weiss 2009: 38). The formation of tooth enamel is also affected by childhood health problems and diseases. Horizontal grooves, known as enamel hypoplasia, present themselves on the canines, incisors, molars, and premolars when the body has undergone stress. They form when the enamel of the crown of the tooth is developing usually between the ages of one and seven. The mineral that forms the crown of the tooth becomes less dense during periods of stress. These lines do not fade with age. They can inform the observer of the general age of the individual when he or she underwent stress because teeth erupt at certain periods in childhood. The width of these lines can indicate a period of prolonged stress, but it is impossible to determine the specific length of time (Mays 1998: 156–61; Weiss 2009: 38).

Similar to enamel hypoplasia, Harris lines form on the long bones, particularly the tibia and shin bones, during periods of stress. Harris lines tend to be faint, and although some can be seen with the naked eye, they are better observed under microscopic and x-ray analysis. They materialize when there was a cessation and resumption of growth in an individual that was caused by an illness or malnutrition. Unlike enamel hypoplasia, they may fade during adulthood. Studies of modern populations of children with poor health have also demonstrated that these lines do not always appear on the bones (Larsen 1997: 40–3; Weiss 2009: 38).

If stresses and strains are noted, the biological anthropologist may also speculate on how one strain on the body might have affected the overall health and movement of an individual. They could also speculate whether the condition might have led to problems later in life, such as arthritis. People often died before reaching old age, so the long-term effects of a condition might never have manifested themselves on the skeletal remains.

A comparative analysis of skeletal remains from different regions and time periods can help to establish whether particular conditions were prevalent in certain regions and/or periods of time. Sometimes demographics are used to see if males, females, or people of different age groups suffered from certain types of strains in comparison to other groups (Weiss 2009: 10–36).

A study of this sort was made by Redfern (2003) who looked closely at the living conditions of women in Roman Britain and the effects urbanism might have had on their health. She found in her samples that women had greater signs of disease and anaemia than men. Her argument was based on a comparison of the skeletal remains with the local environment, and it showed that the living conditions of the individuals along with childbirth and pregnancy were a determining factor in their condition.

7.3.4 Activities

People's activities affect muscular development, which sometimes manifests on the bones. The development of muscles in specific areas of the body can signify possible activities a person may have undertaken during their lifetime. For example, someone who frequently lifted heavy items would develop muscles in their backs and arms. We may be able to recognize that a person had strains or developments that indicate certain activities such as horse riding. However, the bones alone cannot be used to determine *why* the person might have been riding, lifting, or performing an activity. This question might be answered by comparing the skeletal remains with the society to which they belonged. Nonetheless, care must be taken not to juxtapose the skeletal remains with basic and overgeneralized notions of lifestyles in particular places and periods. So caution is advised that when one encounters these forms of interpretation, it is best to question the process by which these observations were arrived (Larsen 1997:161–94).

7.3.5 Status

Sometimes archaeologists will use a person's stature to determine their social status. However, in terms of wealth or power, it is almost impossible to establish status in relation to health. Someone born in squalid conditions might have signs of poor health but have been an emperor, whilst someone born in luxurious conditions with a healthy skeletal frame might have been deemed a social outcast on account of something they did.

Other forms of social status might be determined by signs of activity or conditions of the bones made in comparison to burials. It may be possible to see if those with similar signs of strain were buried in the same manner, with the same objects, or if they were placed together in particular areas of a necropolis. For example, those suffering from certain diseases might have been interred in specific areas of a burial ground. Comparisons such as this can offer new insights into status in relation to bodily condition, but it is almost impossible to determine status in terms of wealth and power based on bodily condition alone.

7.3.6 Diseases

Besides general indicators of stress, some dietary deficiencies and diseases leave traces on bones. These are known as "specific stress indicators" because, unlike the "general stress indicators" mentioned above, it is possible to make a more precise diagnosis of a condition. As always, it is better to make a diagnosis with a complete skeleton because some conditions manifest themselves on various bodily locations.

Vitamin D deficiency, caused mainly by a lack of sunlight, appears on the skeleton in two ways: rickets in subadults and osteomalacia in adults. Rickets is a deformity of the pelvis and lower limbs recognizable through bowed legs. On account of a lack of vitamin D, the bones do not mineralize properly in developing children, and malformations are caused by a lack of weight-bearing ability of the unmineralized hip and leg bones needed to support the upper part of the body. Adults with vitamin D deficiency suffer from osteomalacia visible through curved sacra, unhealed fractures, pelvic deformities, and collapsed vertebral columns. This is rather difficult to diagnose in adults and can be confused with osteopenia or osteoporosis (Mays 1998: 127; Roberts and Cox 2003: 308–10; Weiss 2009: 44–6).

Anaemia, an iron deficiency, is caused by diet, genetic disorders, and parasites which live off blood and use the body as a host for breeding. There are two main features associated with the condition. The first is cribra orbitalia, which consists of small holes that are located on the bone of the inner eye sockets. The second is porotic hyperostosis, which are tiny holes in the skull. Although these indicate anaemia, without aDNA tests, it is sometimes difficult to determine the condition because the signs on the skeleton can be caused by other problems. A comparison with the whole skeleton might provide the anthropologist with a more precise indication of the cause of the anaemia. Childbirth can be a reason, as women can become anaemic when a foetus is developing in the womb. Some parasites that cause the condition can be detected by holes in the bones near the pelvic area (Mays 1998: 142; Weiss 2009: 46–9).

Certain infectious diseases cause the skeleton to mutate, such as tuberculosis, syphilis, and leprosy. Syphilis is a treponemal disease that is divided into four groups: pinta, which has no skeletal markers and is transferred through skin and mucus; yaws, which is transferred through skin and mucus, and destroys the nose and palate of the mouth; endemic syphilis, which is similar to yaws in that it is passed through skin and mucus, and causes the same form of facial destruction; and venereal syphilis, which is passed through sexual contact, and causes the skull, elbows, hips, and knees to deteriorate. Congenital syphilis is passed from a mother to infant through venereal infection, and manifests in dental abnormalities, sometimes indicated with wide gaps between the teeth (Weiss 2009: 52–4).

Mutations caused by leprosy and tuberculosis leave similar traces on the bones that can cause them to be confused in diagnostic examinations. Leprosy is rarely fatal but can disfigure the sufferer. It is generally found in the form of facial and nasal bone destruction and the loss of distal elements, and the bones show no signs of regeneration (Weiss 2009: 56).

Congenital diseases can also be identified on skeletal remains. These are cleft pallet, hydrocephalus, microcephaly, achondroplasia (dwarfism), and club foot. Some of these conditions are severe, and others, such as dwarfism and club foot, are non–life threatening. Severe pathologies are rarely found in the archaeological record because it was likely that infants born with drastic deformities would not have survived, and given the fragility of infant bones, the archaeological record is scarce.

While some of the problems found in the biological archaeological record might not have been noticed or might have been considered only a minor problem when someone was alive, the biological anthropologist might note such problems as a disability. Spina bifida occulta, for example, occurs when the lower sacrum fails to fuse. Since it affects only the lower part of the body, its problems can be minimal if not completely unnoticeable by someone who has the condition. In comparison, the more severe form of spina bifida is cystica, which occurs when the back of the vertebral spine fails to fuse, leaving the spinal nerves unprotected. It often causes foetal death, so it is rare in the archaeological record (Weiss 2009: 60).

Dental diseases are commonly found because the teeth have a strong survival rate in the archaeological record. Most dental conditions show signs of tooth degeneration. Dental attrition, which is general wear on the teeth, can develop over time. In places where the teeth and mouth are used as a tool, attrition may develop more rapidly than in places where this does not occur (Larsen 1997: 254–62). Caries (cavities) are very common in the archaeological record, and range in scale from small enamel opacities to the loss of the tooth crown and roots. They are caused by demineralization of the dental tissue by carbohydrate fermentation (Larsen 1997: 65). Plaque and abscesses are also common on teeth. More serious and debilitating periodontal diseases, such as advanced gingivitis which affects the alveolar bone in the jaw, have been noted in the skeletal record. However, if the condition was only located in the gums, the condition would be invisible on the remains (Larsen 1997: 77).

7.3.7 Trauma and Surgical Procedures

Injuries are represented on bones in forms of fractures, blade, and cut marks. It is extremely difficult to establish an exact cause for most traumas. It might be clear that someone broke a leg, but how they did it may not be determinable. The bone can also indicate whether someone survived a trauma if damage to the bone shows signs of regeneration. Absence of regrowth indicates that the person died of the injury or shortly after it took place.

Injuries are also useful to study because the bones can show signs of surgical treatment. The main procedures that have been identified are trephination, amputation, alignment of fractures, and dental surgery. Tools used in both amputations and trephination can be established because of the types of marks a scalpel or saw would have left on the bone (Start 2002: 114–19).

For the Greek and Roman period, however, the evidence for medical intervention, or published evidence, is slim. Nonetheless, there are a few interesting examples from the Roman period that indicate that some of the procedures described in the medical texts were performed. A foetus discovered at the Roman burial site in Poundbury, Dorest (Molleson and Cox 1988) showed signs of embryotomy or the surgical extraction of a foetus from the womb. The bones are cut in ways that are similarly described by Soranus (*Gyn.* 4.9–14). Yet, it cannot be determined if the infant had died in utero or from the procedure itself. Another example is seen on a thigh bone that was found in a second-century burial outside of Rome. It shows serrated marks left from surgical amputation (Renfrew and Bahn 2008: 458). There is also confirmation that the Romans had the ability to set bones, as some skeletal remains show that broken bones were knit together neatly after the break (Roberts 1988). As for dental surgery, archaeological remains of prosthetic teeth have been found in Etruscan tombs (Becker 1999, 2002).

7.3.8 Retrospective Diagnosis

Biological anthropologists and paleopathologists diagnose the conditions found on the bones they study according to modern medical terms. When they identify a disease or condition, they will speculate how it might have affected the individual's life. However, simply because the diseases can be identified does not mean that those living in the past understood them in the same way as we do in the present. Past treatments, understandings, and attitudes towards bodily conditions may have been quite different from modern conceptions. A modern diagnosis is useful, however, for speculating how the long-term effects of a condition may have influenced the lifestyle of the person who had the problem (Leven 2004). It can be asked, for example, how people with debilitating bone degeneration moved around their environment? Who cared for them? How did they cope with chronic pain? These are all questions that might be considered when a disease is recognized and can be discussed with archaeologists on a wider level to form a rounded understanding of how people dealt with medical conditions in the past.

7.4 ANCIENT DNA ANALYSIS

Difficulties can arise in studies of skeletal remains when the material is incomplete or shows little sign of sexual dimorphism. So in some of these cases, aDNA analysis can be a useful tool for determining sex and some illnesses (Brown 2005: 307–9; Cox 2005: 239; Greene and Moore 2010: 223). In some cases, samples of aDNA have been used to diagnose genetic diseases. Thalassemia, which is the genetic form of anaemia, has been identified. Tuberculosis and malaria also have potential for examination (Brown 2005: 308–9; Roberts and Ingham 2008).

Ancient DNA must be collected from remaining collagen found in the teeth, bones, and skin from inhumed and cremated remains. The DNA can decay over a long period of time, so the technique of extraction requires that the bones be in good condition and, in the case of cremated remains, have not been oxidized (Brown 2005; McKinley and Bond 2005: 287).

Ancient DNA analysis has been in use in archaeology since the late 1980s. However, early studies were prone to contamination with modern DNA, meaning that their results are unreliable (Gearney et al. 2005). Fortunately, the scientific methods have improved since then, and it is becoming an ever more reliable source of information for archaeological use. In spite of all of the advances in aDNA analysis, the problem of contamination with modern DNA is still a risk. It is also a costly exercise, so the studies are only undertaken when a project is well resourced and a need for the analysis can be demonstrated (Brown 2005: 308–9; Roberts and Ingham 2008).

7.5 STABLE ISOTOPE ANALYSIS

A developing field of study in archaeology is stable isotope analysis. Unlike the study of Carbon-14 (^{14}C), which is used in dating organic remains by measuring the breakdown of carbon contained within the remains, stable isotopes of carbon, oxygen, strontium, sulphur, and nitrogen remain constant over time and can tell us about certain aspects of human and animal life in the past. Greene and Moore (2010) provide an introduction to the study of ^{14}C, but to put it simply, ^{14}C is absorbed by all living organisms until they die and then it begins to break down at a fairly regular rate. The technique used in dating measures the radioactivity of an organic sample to find the remaining amount of ^{14}C left in it. The remaining amount of ^{14}C is used to calculate the amount of time that has elapsed from the death of the sample, giving a possible date, though this is never exact (Greene and Moore 2012: 167–76). Carbon-14 is not used to study health-related aspects of a person's life. Stable isotopes can be extracted from collagen, such as aDNA, found in teeth, bones, soft tissues, and hair. Each of the isotopes can be isolated to consider different aspects of past lifestyles that play a role in understanding a person's environment, diet, and migration patterns, all of which could have influenced their health.

Carbon isotopes can provide information about ancient diets and migration patterns. The carbon numbers found in the isotope are variable and dependent upon the types of food the person or animal would have eaten. In general, a diet consisting of marine animals, grasses, and plants can be detected (Sealy 2005: 270–2). This information is useful for helping archaeologists to identify whether an individual might have suffered from a lack of minerals or vitamins in their diets that could have led to conditions such as anaemia. A comparison with other skeletal remains from the same population would make it possible to see if certain problems were widespread and if they were related to their intake or lack of intake of certain foods.

Nitrogen isotopes are found in bone collagen, hair, and muscle. The examination of this isotope is limited to specimens with good collagen preservation. It can be studied like carbon isotopes to determine whether an individual's diet was plant or animal based and, in the case of infants, the age of weaning. Infants who have been breastfed have higher nitrogen levels than their mothers. Their levels begin to decrease as they are being weaned (Sealy 2005: 272–3). Knowing the general age of weaning in a society can also help us to identify when an infant might have gained the socially perceived status of becoming a child in their society.

Oxygen isotopes vary in humans and animals depending on the places from where they originated. This isotope is affected by temperature, altitude, precipitation levels, and distance from the ocean. Oxygen can be found in all human tissue, but it is mainly located in bone phosphate and bone and enamel carbonate. This particular isotope has mainly been used to ascertain migration patterns (Roberts 2009: 205–6; Sealy 2005: 270–6). In relation to health, it might be possible to determine if people who moved into a new population differed in health in comparison to the indigenous skeletal remains. More generally, it can also be used to explain how diseases might have been introduced into a society, given that migration can be a disease vector, as discussed below.

The entire study of isotopes has great potential for future research, but at the moment, there still exists a lack of understanding of how food is converted into body tissue and how these create isotope fractionations. Moreover, this lab-based analysis is expensive, so studies that require examinations of this sort need to be well supported in terms of finance. They also need to be made in laboratories familiar with testing isotopes on ancient remains.

7.6 THE ENVIRONMENT

Having established that the bones are useful archaeological remains for providing information about an individual's health and diet, the focus of this section will describe how archaeologists study ancient environments. The natural environment is studied by some environmental archaeologists in relation to disease ecology. This is a specific area of archaeological science that is concerned with establishing the natural living conditions people would have been exposed to in their lifetimes that influenced their overall health and well-being (Ortner 2005: 225–33). The environment in which we live is filled with infectious organisms and toxic materials that influence our growth and development. Additionally, surrounding environments sometime lack substances that are necessary for the maintenance of health, such as a fresh supply of water and a varied diet consisting of fresh foods. When these are lacking, humans adapt their surroundings to ensure their survival, such as building irrigation ditches in arid regions to facilitate agricultural development. When changes such as this are implemented, the surrounding natural environment might change. For example, an irrigation system will not only alter the appearance of the landscape but also allows for new forms of vegetation and fauna (including insects) to appear. People may develop allergic reactions to newly introduced plants because they do not have an immunity to foreign pollens, insects may carry new diseases, and diets would have changed in accordance to what was grown (Ortner 2005: 225).

7.6.1 Ascertaining Past Environments

To ascertain what a past environment was like, environmental archaeologists consider temperature ranges, average rainfalls, and temporary changes in local environments caused by unusual events, such as volcanic activity. They look for signs of the environments in soil samples, which contain the remains of seeds, pollens, and invertebrates, such as snails and mites. These not only let them know what types of flora and fauna were common in a region, but also give an idea of temperature and levels of rainfall, since plants and invertebrates survive in particular conditions (Evans and O'Connor 1999: 132–47). The process of flotation is used to retrieve this information from the soil. This involves placing a soil sample in a bucket or container with holes in the bottom. When the bucket is submerged about halfway into water, it is agitated to loosen the soil. The heavier stones and silt will sink to the bottom of the container, while the seeds, pollens, small bones, particularly those of fish and fowl, will float to the top of the container. These are then examined under a microscope for identification by entomologists, biological anthropologists, and palaeobotanists.

Surviving samples of trees can also inform the environmental archaeologist about past landscapes. Variations in tree-ring width give us an indication of climatic conditions in particular years – a moist year will yield wider tree rings than those in a dry year (Evans and O'Conner 1999: 132–47; Greene and Moore 2010: 192–205; Renfrew and Bahn 2008: 231–74).

For disease ecologists, knowing the climatic conditions can also help determine what diseases might have been common in a region. They can compare the climate with skeletal remains to see if there is a link in bodily condition with diseases common to specific areas. The study of malaria is a good example of this type of examination. This disease is and was found in places that are warm and moist which can support the anopheles mosquitos responsible for spreading the *Plasmodium* genus of a protozoan parasite that causes malaria (Roberts and Cox: 2003: 170). The identification of the mosquito in soil samples by a palaeoentomologist – someone who examines the remains of insects – can help to determine whether there was a vector for the disease in the area being studied. Although malaria does not affect the skeleton, it sometimes causes anaemia, which, as described, does leave traces on bones. It is now possible to detect malaria through aDNA analysis (Taylor,

Rutland, and Molleson 1997). Therefore, comparisons between environments, archaeological sites, and the remains of bodies help to locate places common for particular diseases.

7.6.2 Localized Diets and Living Conditions

Besides climate, on a more localized scale, environmental archaeologists can also consider various types of living conditions to gain a wide perspective of what life was like in particular places in the past, such as urban or rural areas. Plant and animal remains, usually found through a study of soil samples taken from hearths and areas where domestic waste might have been discarded, are examined in these instances. The seeds, butchered bones, and pollens located in these contexts can also help to show which foods might have been imported, hunted, gathered from the natural environment, or raised as domesticated crops and animals.

A recent study by van der Veen (2011) has identified food and medicinal plants that were traded at the Roman and Islamic ports of Quseir al-Qadim, Egypt. Once a food is recognized, consideration is given to storage, trade, and growing seasons because these aspects all play a role in determining the quantity and quality of food available to people at specific times of the year (Ortner 2005: 227). If a food and/or medicinal product is found to have been imported, archaeologists can then ask why certain products were popular. There could be many answers to this question, such as a general appreciation for certain foods or perhaps a belief that ingredients from certain areas were better for one's health or made more effective medicines.

Diets can also be accessed by food remains found in the intestines of mummified bodies and coprolites (dried human excrement) and faecal matter (usually found in cesspits and latrine drains). The remains can contain fibrous matter: small bones, scales, skin, meat, hair, plant fibres, pollens, and seeds (Greene and Moore 2010: 221). Sometimes there is evidence for people having eaten imported foods through seeds found in the waste. Intestinal parasites are also found in these types of remains (Holden 2005: 403–5).

Animal bones, both wild and domestic, are also indicative of diet. Bones used in cooking will sometimes show signs of butchering and burning (Greene and Moore 2010: 205–14; O'Connor 2004; Renfrew and Bahn 2008: 291–301). Sometimes coprolites contain the remains of insects, indicating that people were also ingesting bugs as part of their diet (Robinson 2005: 131). The remains of animals found on archaeological sites also help in revealing what types of animals were raised for food or kept for by-products such as milk, and/or used for the production of their skin and hair. Sheep, for example, are useful for milk, wool, the production of lamb, and can be eaten as mutton. Archaeologists can generally identify the species and often whether it was a wild or domesticated creature. From this information, it is possible to ascertain whether a group of people preferred a diet of hunted or domesticated creatures. In some instances, it is not always possible to determine whether the animal was domesticated or wild, particularly in the case of dogs or cats.

When studying local environments, the archaeologist can often determine what living conditions might have been like. The study made by Redfern (2003), discussed above, also compared the skeletal remains to evidence for living conditions in urban areas of Roman Britain. She found that the conditions were not hygienic by modern standards. The environmental and entomological studies made at the site in 1 Poultry, London, showed that the walls of the houses had signs of head lice, which implies an endemic problem of infestation. Animals were kept in gardens by the house and the water supply, and this can mean their waste was a potential contaminate. Moreover, a number of houses were close to industrial areas for tanning, and this could have allowed run-off water to enter the water supply.

In Ostia and Pompeii, latrines have been found by the kitchen. Although strange or repulsive to modern sentiment, to the archaeologist, this proximity can suggest that there was a lack of distinction concerning household waste. Human and food waste alike could be discarded in the same area. This indicates that there are social/cultural views on places where waste was to be discarded and what we see as an unhygienic practice. Romans were likely unaware that flies feasting on waste and landing on food would most likely pass on parasite eggs, germs, and diseases.

7.6.3 Disease Vectors

Animals are also studied to determine whether they were vectors (carriers) of diseases to which people might have been exposed. Wild animal bones found in domestic contexts, such as rats and mice, can indicate the possible spread of epidemic diseases, such as plague. Domesticated animals such as dogs, cats, sheep, and pigs commonly contract intestinal worms and other parasites that can be passed to humans. These will appear in the human skeleton as small holes in bones where the larvae of the parasite of the worm will develop. This disease is known as echinococcosis (Ortner 2005: 230–2). Diseases can also be passed from wild animals to domesticated animals and ultimately to the human population. A good example of this chain is found in tuberculosis, which can originate in wild animals, is passed to cattle, and then to humans

(Roberts and Buikstra 2003). Insects also carry disease, as discussed above with malaria, and the study of their remains can help us further to ascertain the possible disease vectors in past environments.

Population size and human migration contribute to the spread of illness as well. If people lived in close proximity to one another, then there is the possibility for diseases or disease outbreaks to spread quickly throughout a community. Thus, an examination of urban and rural layouts, housing, and local amenities (discussed in the previous chapter) can be employed to note where waste and sewage were disposed in relation to dwelling areas.

Migration can also facilitate the spread of diseases. Although we have written records about people's migration, another way to determine how people moved is to look at the oxygen isotope that is found in their remains. Movement between places can introduce new pathogens to areas, especially where people may not have had immunity to a disease.

7.7 ARCHAEOBOTANICAL REMAINS AND RESIDUE SAMPLES

Although environmental archaeologists will look for plant remains to determine the landscape and types of crops grown in an area, they can also make smaller-scale studies to determine what plants might have been stored in containers or used in medicines. Writers such as Pliny the Elder, the Hippocratic writers, Dioscorides, and Theophrastus described the ingredients used in ancient pharmaceutical remedies (Scarborough 1977, 1978, 1983, 2010; Totelin 2009). Even though they might have recommended specific plants, minerals, and animals in their recipes, we cannot be certain if doctors or pharmacists in the Greco-Roman world followed their advice unless we examine archaeological remains, which can be found in soil samples from Roman house gardens, the residues left in pottery, and the rare examples of surviving medicines in the archaeological record. Taking soil samples from known gardens can indicate the types of plants grown around a domestic site, and these can be compared to the ancient medical texts. However, even if certain plants mentioned in these sources are identified, it cannot be assumed that they were strictly used for their medicinal properties. The majority of ingredients mentioned in ancient texts could have been used in a number of ways, such as for food, make-up, paints, inks, decoration, and clothing dyes.

Plant, animal, and insect remains are sometimes found in ancient containers, which might help in the identification of medicines. For example, some plant remains were found in *dolia* (large vats partially placed in the ground, used for storing food), in the cellar of a Roman villa rustica, the

Villa Vesuvio, in Scafati, near Pompeii. One of the *dolia* had a waterlogged deposit of organic material that contained seeds, plant remains, and reptile and amphibian bones. Ciaraldi (1997, 2000, 2002) argued that the presence of a particular type of cooker found near the containers also helped to support her interpretation that this was an area for drug preparation. She then compared the botanical and animal remains to Dioscorides and Pliny the Elder, and noted that the remains mentioned in the texts were also found in the containers (Ciaraldi 1997, 2000, 2002). It is possible that she is correct, but there needs to be more studies made on the production of medicinal ingredients to see if this was done at a household level in the ancient world, much like medieval physic gardens. Alternatively, people may have bought medicines from special shops.

On a microscopic level, residue samples from pottery vessels that might have been used for storing medicines can also be studied to determine what ingredients were stored in the vessels. This examination involves the identification of lipids, which are animal fats, plant oils, waxes, and resins. In comparison to aDNA, carbohydrates, proteins, and lipids survive quite well in the archaeological record. Vessels are examined at the molecular level to match molecules found in specific flora and fauna. The process is made through gas chromatography, which separates the different lipids found within a sample. Sometimes this is combined with mass spectrometry, which gives more precise molecular structural information of different lipids. This is particularly useful when only traces of a material exist (Evershed et al. 2005: 331). As with plants found in gardens, when residue samples are taken, an important question to ask is whether the container was used specifically to hold medicines. In certain cases, pottery remains might have the name of a medicine stamped on it, which makes it easier to compare the mixture with textual sources to see if the recipe suggested in the literature was followed in practice.

Sometimes the actual medicines survive. There is a case from Lyon where Roman *collyria* (sticks of eye medicine) were found with the names of the medicines stamped on them. Interestingly, the names of the remedies could be matched to ancient texts, and it was found that the ingredients used in the medicines did not match the ingredients recommended in the recipe. This is a significant find because it showed that the textual sources do not always correspond with the archaeological evidence. Thus, it needs to be asked why Roman terms were used for medicines if the ingredients varied. Since these were found in Gaul, it may have been that local or more easily available ingredients were substituted for ones that the doctor/pharmacist could not obtain. It has been suggested that perhaps the Latin terms for the ingredients were not understood. In such instances, a different ingredient may have been substituted, or perhaps it was the Roman name that was important for selling medicines rather than the ingredients (Boyer 1990).

Archaeobotany is also useful for identifying trade in ingredients. If a plant, mineral, or animal was not indigenous, then one needs to ask about the trade and the costs involved with importing materials (van der Veen 2011). This not only gives us information about trade, but also allows us to consider whether foreign materials were believed to have been more efficacious because of their exoticness.

7.8 METAL, CERAMIC, AND WOOD ANALYSIS

The study of ceramic petrology can be used to see if pottery vessels were made in particular areas of the Greco-Roman world. As a means of noting origin, thin slices of pottery are often examined under a microscope to match the minerals found in the pottery to a region (Henderson 2000: 11–13). In a combined study of residue or botanical remains found in pottery, one could possibly use ceramic petrology to determine if ceramics from a certain area or type were considered best for the storage of certain ingredients.

Wood can also be studied for its place of origin. This can be important when examining votive offerings of body parts that have been found in waterlogged locations, such as those found in Gaul (Detys 1988). If the type of wood identified was local to the area, one can ask if there was a functional and/or ritual significance to the type of wood being used in the production of votive body parts (as discussed in Chapter 5).

Many medical instruments are constructed of a copper alloy or bronze, and sometimes it is possible to analyse where the raw materials used in the fabrication of medical tools originated. Having access to this information can help us learn about Greco-Roman trade in metals. The metals are usually studied through metallography, when a thin section of the metal is examined under a microscope. The section of metal also has to be polished and etched in order to see structural differences to determine the composition of metals (Greene and Moore 2010: 229). Following on from this analysis, one can ask whether the raw material for medical tools came from one area and why this might have been. In comparison to the ancient literature, Galen (2.682K), for example, says the best metal for scalpel blades came from the province of Noricum, in what is now Austria. Although this might have been true, we as medical historians should ask if this was simply the opinion of Galen or if other doctors concurred.

Tests on some metals, copper alloys for example, are possible to make to determine from where the raw materials originated (Hurcombe 2007:

194–202). Steel, on the other hand, cannot be studied for its place of origin (Hurcombe 2007: 205). Nonetheless, in reference to Galen, there is archaeological evidence for steel production in Noricum. Iron carbonate from the region yields steel when it is smelted because it contains manganese which creates an alloy. Three- to six-foot shaft furnaces for the production of steel have been found in the province (Cech 2008), so it is possible that the province was known for its metal, and Galen might have been aware of this.

The place of origin for bronze and copper can be found through a range of metal analyses of the raw materials, but this does not indicate where the objects were made. Raw materials can be transported long distances, indicated by archaeological remains of shipwrecks carrying bronze ingots, for example. Since it is possible to determine the origin of copper alloys, this information can be used to study the distribution of the materials and/or medical instruments throughout the Roman world.

If it became apparent that materials from particular areas were commonly used in the production of objects used for medical practices, then an archaeologist could question the ease of trade and access to the natural resource. It can also be asked if some materials were perceived to have had particular healing powers, as seen with the properties of stone and other medical ingredients.

7.9 USE-WEAR AND BLOOD ANALYSES ON TOOLS

Studying metals also allows the archaeologist to see how the objects were made and gives an insight into the technologies used in the production of them. For instance, it can be determined if an object was hammered, smelted, or cold smelted, any of which might provide us with an understanding of local techniques of design. Through microscopic examinations of cutting edges, it is also possible to determine how objects were used. The focus of use-wear analysis (Greene and Moore 2010: 229) has tended to centre on flint blades from the prehistoric periods, but it can also be applied to other objects that were used in cutting. Hence, it might be possible to see if blades on surgical tools were used to cut bone. In an ideal situation, the archaeological context of the tools would be known and the cutting edges would have survived. In such cases, comparisons could be made to see if objects with no signs of use had other functions such as votive offerings, particularly if they were found in a ritual context.

Along with studying the blades for signs of use, recent developments in forensics have made it possible to find blood on objects. This type of study was developed in the 1980s with the intention of attempting to locate the remains of blood on flint tools in order to determine the types of animals that were butchered in prehistoric periods. Nonetheless, one of the main problems with the technique is that the blood can become contaminated both by those working in the lab and from its condition of being deposited in soil for thousands of years.

One of the most recent techniques that could be used for the study of blood is DNA in blood residue analysis. DNA analysis is formed by using the polymerase chain reaction (PCR). This involves taking a piece of DNA and producing a chain of up to a million copies of the same pieces. This means that where little blood exists, a larger sample of the DNA strand will be created and then the species can be identified (Smith and Wilson 2005: 319–20). The techniques are still in their infancy, but if blood can be gathered from medical tools, it might be possible to tell if they were used on animals, humans, or possibly both. Moreover, some tools do not seem to have been found in the medical contexts such as in areas known for leather working or in burials. Thus checking for blood and/or use could help to identify a function of the objects.

7.10 CONCLUSION

The subjects discussed in this chapter show the variety of methods for examining remains that require a scientific or anatomical knowledge and are therefore undertaken by specialists. The information yielded from these examinations can then be used to ask questions about the health and diet of people living in the past, and can be compared with archaeological contexts of objects and landscapes. They allow for a broader approach to past remains. However, some of the studies are in their infancy or require a large sample of materials to make a viable study. Nonetheless, there is potential from these methods to enhance our awareness of past medical practices, health, and pharmaceutical remains in the Greco-Roman world.

CONSIDERATION QUESTIONS

1. Consider how the methods mentioned in this chapter might be used in relation to ancient medical texts?
2. What information might these scientific studies reveal to us about medicine in the past?

FURTHER READING

Andrews, K., and R. Doonan 2003. *Test Tubes and Trowels: Using Science in Archaeology*. Stroud: Tempus.

Aufderheide, A. C., and C. Rodríguez-Martín 1998. *The Cambridge Encyclopaedia of Human Paleopathology*. Cambridge: Cambridge University Press.

Brothewell, D. R., and A. M. Pollard, eds. 2005. *Handbook of Archaeological Sciences*. Chichester: John Wiley.

Roberts, C. A., and K. Manchester 2005. *The Archaeology of Disease*. Stroud: Sutton.

Roberts, C. A., and M. Cox 2003. *Health and Disease in Britain: From Prehistory to the Present Day*. Stroud: Sutton.

Weiss, E. 2009. *Bioarchaeological Science: What We Have Learned from Human Skeletal Remains*. New York: Nova Science.

Wilkinson, K., and C. Stevens 2005. *Environmental Archaeology: Approaches, Techniques and Applications*. Stroud: Tempus.

CHAPTER 8

CONCLUSION

It was mentioned in Chapter 1 that one of the hindrances to interdisciplinary studies is the way in which scholars do not make their fields of study relevant to people who specialize in different subjects. The main point of this book was to remedy one version of this impasse by introducing archaeological methods and theories of enquiry to medical historians. The subject of Greco-Roman medical history is stimulating. It introduces us to the manners in which people perceived their bodies and treatments, and maintained their health. Yet because we tend to think ancient history is primarily accessed through its literary sources, we tend not to think what significant details about everyday life the texts may be omitting. The examination of material remains can therefore greatly enhance our awareness of conceptions of the body and health, forms of treatments, and social rules concerning the use, construction, and function of medical objects and spaces in the Greco-Roman world. Without a study of material remains, we would not know if some conceptions of ancient medicine mentioned in the philosophical texts were pervasive in ancient societies. We would not have access to how the majority of people living in the ancient world, who probably did not read or write, practiced and understood medicine. It is the archaeological remains that ultimately give the "silent majority" a voice – a voice that sometimes tells us very different stories to those found in the extant medical literature.

Yet as we have seen, understanding and interpreting archaeological remains is not a straightforward task. Therefore, to make the reader aware of how studies of an archaeological nature are undertaken, each of the main chapters dealt with three core issues. The first issue centred on different debates in the field of archaeology and history to demonstrate the changing nature, developments, and issues that concern researchers undertaking investigations of material remains. The second issue involved the demonstration of the fundamental procedures and questions that need to be addressed when examining the different types of material. The third issue discussed the types of questions and information that can be derived from the remains in order to enhance our awareness of medicine in the past. As these three issues were explained with the use of medically related examples, it is my hope that the reader – medical historian or emerging archaeologist – will now have the basic knowledge to use and/or critically judge, archaeological information for themselves.

Although archaeology is not an easy subject and requires critical attention to detail, it *is* exciting. It forces us to think creatively about the subject of ancient medicine in new and innovative ways that can even challenge our own preconceptions. If, after reading this book, students and scholars of medical history are inclined to use and think about archaeological remains in their work, then the aim of the book has been achieved. If a reader, who never thought he or she would have an interest in archaeology, decides to join an excavation, then may your trowel never dull!

BIBLIOGRAPHY

PRIMARY SOURCES

Albucasis *On Surgery and Instruments: A Definitive Edition of the Arabic Text with English Translation and Commentary*, M. S. Spink and G. L. Lewis, trans., 1973. London: Wellcome Institute of the History of Medicine.

Aristophanes *Wealth*. J. Henderson, trans., 1998–2007. Cambridge, MA: Harvard University Press (Loeb).

Aristotle *Metaphysics*. J. Sachs, trans., 2002. Santa Fe, NM: Green Lion Press.

Celsus *De Medicina*. W. G. Spencer, trans., 1971. Cambridge, MA: Harvard University Press (Loeb).

Dionysius of Halicarnassus. E. Carey, trans., 1947. Cambridge, MA: Harvard University Press (Loeb).

Dioscorides. Pedanius Dioscorides of Anazarbus, *De Materia Medica*. L. Beck, trans., 2005. Hildesheim: Olms-Weidmann.

Frontinus *The Aqueducts of Rome*. C. E. Bennet and C. L. Herschel, trans., and M. McElwain, ed., 1980. Cambridge, MA: Harvard University Press (Loeb).

Galen *Claudii Galeni opera omnia*. C. G. Kühn, ed., 20 vols. in 22. 1821–1833. Leipzig: Cnobloch.

    On Consolation from Grief (Peri Alupesias, Ne Pas se Chagriner). V. Boudon-Millot and J. Jouanna, trans. and eds., 2010. Paris: Les Belles Lettres (Budé).

    Hygiene (de Sanitate tuenda). R. M. Green, trans., 1951. Springfield, IL: Charles C. Thomas.

Herodotus *Histories*. A. Godley, trans., 1963. Cambridge, MA: Harvard University Press (Loeb).

Hippocrates *Airs Waters Places*. W. H. S. Jones, trans., 1953. London: William Heinemann (Loeb).

    Canon. W. H. S. Jones, trans., 1953. London: William Heinemann (Loeb).

    Decorum. W. H. S. Jones, trans., 1953. London: William Heinemann (Loeb).

    In the Surgery. W. H. S. Jones, trans., 1953. London: William Heinemann (Loeb).

    The Nature of Man. W. H. S. Jones, trans., 1953. London: William Heinemann (Loeb).

    The Physician. W. H. S. Jones, trans., 1953. London: William Heinemann (Loeb).

Hyginus *Liber de Munitionibus Castrorum*. W. Gemoll, ed., 1897. Leipzig: B. G. Teubner.

Livy *Ab Urbe Condita*, Vols. I and II. C. F. Walters and R. S. Conway, eds., 1974 (I); 1919 (II). Oxford: Clarendon Press.

Lucian *The Ignorant Book Collector (Adversus Indoctum)*. A. M. Harmon, trans., 1921. London: William Heinemann Press (Loeb).

    Philopseudes. A. M. Harmon, trans., 1921. London: William Heinemann Press (Loeb).

Martial *Epigrams*. D. R. Shackleton Bailey, trans., 1993. Cambridge, MA: Harvard University Press (Loeb).

Ovid *Metamorphoses* 2 vols. F. J. Miller, trans., 1960, 1966. Cambridge, MA: Harvard University Press (Loeb).

Paul of Aegina. *Paulus Aegineta*. I. L. Heiberg, ed., 1921–4. Leipzig: B. G. Teubner.

Pausanias *Description of Greece*. W. H. S. Jones, trans., 1959. Cambridge, MA: Harvard University Press (Loeb).

Plato *The Republic*. Paul Shorey, trans., 1956. London: William Heinemann (Loeb).

Pliny *Natural History*. H. Rackham, trans., 1960. Cambridge, MA: Harvard University Press (Loeb).

Plutarch *Moralia*. F. C. Babbit, trans., 1960. Cambridge, MA: Harvard University Press (Loeb).

Scriptores Historiae Augustae. D. Magie, trans., 1921–1932. London: William Heinemann Press (Loeb).

Soranus *Gynecology*. O. Temkin, trans., 1956. Baltimore, MD: Johns Hopkins University Press.

Strabo *Geography* 2 vols. H. L. Jones, trans. 1960/1969. Cambridge, MA: Harvard University Press (Loeb).

Suetonius *The Lives of the Twelve Caesars*. J. C. Rolfe, trans., 1959. Cambridge, MA: Harvard University Press (Loeb).

Tacitus *Germania* 1959. Cambridge, MA: Harvard University Press (Loeb).

Theophrastus *Enquiry into Plants* 2 vols. A. Hort, trans., 1961. Cambridge, MA: Harvard University Press (Loeb).

Vegetius *Epitome of Military Science*. N. P. Milner, trans., 1996. Liverpool: Liverpool University Press.

Virgil *Aeneid*. R. D. Williams, ed., 1973. London: MacMillen.

Vitruvius *On Architecture* 2 vols. F. Granger, trans., 1962. Cambridge, MA: Harvard University Press (Loeb).

CATALOGUES MENTIONED IN THE TEXT

AE   *L'Année Épigraphique: Revue des Publications Épigraphiques Relatives à l'antiquité Romaine.* 1888 Paris.

BGU   *Berliner Griechische Urkunden Ägyptische Urkunden aus den Königlichen Museen zu Berlin.* 1895 Berlin.

BMC   *British Museum Catalogue of Greek Coins*, Vols. 1–29. London: British Museum Press.

BMC   RE Mattingly, H. 1923–1975 *Coins of the Roman Empire in the British Museum*, Vols. 1–6.

CIG   *Corpus Inscriptionum Graecarum*. Berlin: Könliglich Preussische Akademie der Wissenschaften zu Berlin.

CIL   *Corpus Inscriptionum Latinorum. Consilio et Ductoritate Academie Litterarum Regiae Borussical Edition*. Berlin: Academieder Wissenschaften 1862.

Crawford, M. H. 1974. *Roman Republican Coinage*, Vols. 1–2. Cambridge: Cambridge University Press.

CVA   *Corpus Vasorum Antiquorum*. http://www.cvaonline.org

Grueber, H. A., and Poole, R. S. 1910. *Coins of the Roman Republic in the British Museum*, Vols. 1–3. London: British Museum.

IG   *Inscriptiones Graecae*. Berlin: Brandenburgische Akademie der Wissenschaften.

IGRR   *Inscriptiones Graecae ad res Romanas pertinentes: Auctoritate et Impensis Academiae Inscriptionum et litterarum humaniarum*. Rome: L'Erma Bretschneider.

ILS   *Inscriptiones Latinae Selectae*. H. Dessau 1892–1916. Berlin: Apud Weidmannos.

LIMC   *Lexicon Iconographicum Mythologiae Classicae*. 1981–1997. Zürich: Artemis Verlag.

Mattingly, H. et al. 1923–1981. *The Roman Imperial Coinage*, Vols. 1–9. London: Spink.

PGM   H. D. Betz, ed. 1996. *The Greek Magical Papyri in Translation: Including Demotic Spells*. Chicago: University of Chicago Press.

P.Mich.   *Papyri in the University of Michigan Collection*. Ann Arbor: University of Michigan Press

P.Oxy   *The Oxyrhynchus Papyri.* B. Grenfell, A. S. Hunter et al., eds. 1898 London.

P. Rainer   *Papyrus Erzherzog Rainer der Papyrussammlung der Österreichischen Nationalbibliothek.*
              Vienna: Verlag Brüder Hollinek 1883

RIB   *The Roman Inscriptions of Britain.* R. G. Collingwood and R. P. Wright, eds. 1995.
              Stroud: Alan Sutton.

SECONDARY SOURCES

Aicher, P. J. 1995. *Guide to the Aqueducts of Ancient Rome.* Wauconda, IL: Bolchazy-Carducci.

Aleshire, S. B. 1989. *The Athenian Askelpieion: The People, Their Dedication and Their Inventories.*
    Amsterdam: Gieben.

Allison, P. 1997. "Why do Excavation Reports Have Finds' Catalogues?" In *Not so Much a Pot,
    More a Way of Life,* C. G. Cumberpatch and P. W. Blinkhorn, eds. Oxbow Monograph 83.
    Oxford: Oxbow Books, pp. 77–84.

    1999a. "Introduction". In *The Archaeology of Household Activities,* P. Allison, ed. London:
    Routledge, pp. 1–18.

    1999b. "Labels for Ladles: Interpreting the Material Culture of Roman Households", In *The
    Archaeology of Household Activities,* P. Allison, ed. London: Routledge, pp. 57–77.

Alvarez Sáenz de Buruaga, J. 1945. "Museo Arqueológico de Mérida (Badajoz)", *Memoires de los
    Museos Arqueologico Provinciales* 6: 4–10.

Alvarez Sáenz de Buruaga, J., and J. García de Soto 1946. "Nuevas aportacioines al estudio de
    la Necrópolis Oriental de Mérida", *Archivo Español de Arqueología* 19: 70–85.

Anderson, R. 2002. "Kill or Cure: Athenian Judicial Curses and the Body in Fear". In *Practitioners,
    Practices and Patients New Approaches to Medical Archaeology and Anthropology: Conference Proceedings,*
    P. Baker and G. Carr, eds. Oxford: Oxbow Books, pp. 221–35.

Andorlini, I., ed. 1997. *Specimina per il Corpus dei papyri greci di medicina: atti dell'Inconto di studio,
    Firenze, 28–29 Marzo 1996.* Florence: G. Vitelli.

    2001–. *Greek Medical Papyri.* Florence: G. Vitelli.

Andrews, K., and R. Doonan 2003. *Test Tubes and Trowels: Using Science in Archaeology.* Stroud:
    Tempus.

Argyle, M. 1988. *Bodily Communication.* London: Routledge.

Ashmore, W., and A. B. Knapp, eds. 1999. *Archaeologies of Landscape.* Oxford: Blackwell.

Aufderheide, A. C., and C. Rodríguez-Martín 1998. *The Cambridge Encyclopaedia of Human
    Paleopathology.* Cambridge: Cambridge University Press.

Baatz, D. 1970. "Krankenhauser bei den Römern", *Kurz und Gut* 2: 8–10.

Bagnall, R., ed. 2009. *The Oxford Handbook of Papyrology.* Oxford: Oxford University Press.

Bahn, P., ed. 1992. *Collins Dictionary of Archaeology.* Glasgow: Harper Collins.

Baker, P. 2002a. "Diagnosing Some Ills: The History and Archaeology of Roman Medicine".
    In *Practitioners, Practices and Patients New Approaches to Medical Archaeology and Anthropology:
    Conference Proceedings,* P. Baker and G. Carr, eds. Oxford: Oxbow Books, pp. 16–29.

    2002b. "The Roman Military Valetudinaria: Fact or Fiction". *The Archaeology of Medicine Papers
    Given at the Session of the Annual Conference of the Theoretical Archaeology Group Held at the University
    of Birmingham on 20 December 1998,* R. Arnott, ed. Oxford: British Archaeological Reports
    International Series 1046, pp. 69–80.

    2004a. *Medical Care for the Roman Army on the Rhine, Danube and British Frontiers from the First through
    Third Centuries AD.* British Archaeological Reports International Series 1286. Oxford:
    Hadrian Books.

    2004b. "Roman Medical Instruments: Archaeological Interpretations of their Possible
    'Non-functional' Uses", *Social History of Medicine* 17: 3–21.

    2011. "Collyrium Stamps: An Indicator of Regional Medical Practices in Roman Gaul",
    European Journal of Archaeology 14(1–2): 158–89.

    2012. "Medieval Islamic Hospitals: Structural Design and Social Perceptions". In *Medicine and
    Space: Body, Surroundings and Borders in Antiquity and the Middle Ages,* P. Baker, H. Nijdam, and
    C. van 't Land, eds. Leiden: Brill, pp. 245–72.

Baker, P., H. Nijdam, and C. van 't Land, eds. 2012. *Medicine and Space: Body, Surroudings and Borders in Antiquity and the Middle Ages*. Leiden: Brill.

Barefoot, P. 2005. "Buildings for Health: Then and Now". In *Health in Antiquity*, H. King, ed. London: Routledge, pp. 205–15.

Barker, P. 1986. *Understanding Archaeological Excavations*. London: B. T. Batsford.

2002. *Techniques of Archaeological Excavation*. London: Routledge.

Barrett, J. 1993. *Fragments from Antiquity: Archaeology of Social Life in Britain 2900–1200 BC*. Oxford: Blackwell.

Beard, M. 1985. "Writing and Ritual: A Study of Diversity and Expansion in the Arval Archive", *Papers of the British School at Rome* 53: 114–32.

Beard, M., and J. Henderson 2001. *Classical Art from Greece to Rome*. Oxford: Oxford University Press.

Becker, M. J. 1999. "Etruscan Gold Dental Appliances: Three Newly 'Discovered' Examples", *American Journal of Archaeology* 103(1): 103–11.

2002. "Etruscan Female Tooth Evulsion: Gold Dental Appliances as Ornaments". In *Practitioners, Practices and Patients New Approaches to Medical Archaeology and Anthropology: Conference Proceedings*, P. Baker and G. Carr, eds. Oxford: Oxbow Books, pp. 238–59.

Bender, B. 1993. "Introduction: Landscape – Meaning and Action". In *Landscape: Politics and Perspectives*, B. Bender, ed. Oxford: Berg, pp. 1–17.

1998. *Stonehenge Making Space*. Oxford: Berg.

Berger, A. A. 2009. *What Objects Mean: An Introduction to Material Culture*. Walnut Creek, CA: West Coast Press.

Binford, L. R. 1962. "Archaeology as Anthropology", *American Antiquity* 28(2): 217–26.

1972. *An Archaeological Perspective*. New York: Seminar Press.

Bintliff, J., and M. Pearce, eds. 2011. *The Death of Archaeological Theory*. Oxford: Oxbow Books.

Blake, E. 2007. "Space, Spatiality, and Archaeology". In *A Companion to Social Archaeology*, L. Meskell and R. W. Preucel, eds. Oxford: Blackwell, pp. 230–54.

Bliquez, L. 1981a. "An Unidentified Roman Surgical Instrument in Bingen", *Journal of the History of Medicine* 36(2): 219–20.

1981b. "Greek and Roman Medicine", *Archaeology* 34(2): 10–17.

1992. "The Hercules Motif on Greco-Roman Surgical Tools". In *From Epidaurus to Salerno: Symposium held at the European University Centre for Cultural Heritage, Ravello, April 1990*, A. Krug, ed. Rixenstart, Belgium: PACT 34, pp. 35–50.

1994. *Roman Surgical Implements and Other Minor Objects in the National Archaeological Museum of Naples*. Mainz: Verlag Philipp von Zabern.

Bliquez, L., and J. P. Oleson 1994. "The Origins, Early History and Applications of the *Pyoulkos* (syringe)". In *Science et Vie Intellectuelle à Alexandrie*, G. Argoud, ed. Saint-Étienne: Publications de l'Université de Saint-Étienne, pp. 83–103.

Boardman, J. 1978. *Greek Sculpture: The Archaic Period*. London: Thames and Hudson.

1985. *Greek Sculpture: The Classical Period*. London: Thames and Hudson.

1996 (4th ed.). *Greek Art*. London: Thames and Hudson.

Bodel, J. 2001. "Epigraphy and the Ancient Historian". In *Epigraphic Evidence: Ancient History from Inscriptions*, J. Bodel, ed. London: Routledge, pp. 1–56.

Boon, G. 1983. "Potters, Oculists and Eye Troubles", *Britannia* 14: 1–12.

Borobia Melendo, E. L. 1988. *Instrumental medico-quirurgico en la hispania romana*. Madrid: Impressos Numancia.

Bourdieu, P. 1973. "The Berber House". In *Rules and Meanings*, M. Douglas, ed. Harmondsworth: Penguin Education, pp. 98–110.

1977. *Outline of the Theory of Practice*, R. Nice, trans. Cambridge: Cambridge University Press.

Bowen Ward, R. 1992. "Women in Roman Baths", *Harvard Theological Revue* 85: 125–47.

Bowman, A. K., and J. D. Thomas 1974. *The Vindolanda Writing Tablets*. Newcastle upon Tyne: Frank Graham.

1991. "A Military Strength Report from Vindolanda", *Journal of Roman Studies* 81: 62–73.

1994. *The Vindolanda Writing Tablets (Tabulae Vindolandenses II)*. London: British Museum Press.

Bowman, A. K. , J. D. Thomas, and R. S. O. Tomlin 2011. "The Vindolanda Writing-Tablets (Tabulae *Vindolandenses* IV, Part 2)", *Britannia* 42: 113–44.

Boyer, R. 1990. "Découverte de la tombe d'un oculiste à Lyon", *Gallia* 47: 215–49.

Brat, L. 1966. *Die Geschichte des Peter Friedrich Ludwigs Hospitals (1841–1966)*. Oldenburg: G. Stalling.

Brendel, O. J. 1979. *Prolegomena to the Study of Roman Art*. New Haven, CT: Yale University Press.

Brown, T. A. 2005. "Ancient DNA". In *Handbook of Archaeological Sciences*, D. R. Brothwell and A. M. Pollard, eds. Chichester: John Wiley, pp. 295–300.

Buchli, V. 2002. "Introduction". In *The Material Culture Reader*, V. Buchli, ed. Oxford: Berg, pp. 1–22.

Bülow-Jacobsen, A. 2009. "Writing Materials in the Ancient World". In *The Oxford Handbook of Papyrology*, R. Bagnall, ed. Oxford: Oxford University Press, pp. 3–29.

Butler, J. 1999. *Gender Trouble: Feminism and the Subversion of Identity*. London: Routledge.

Caldwell, J. 1959. "The New American Archaeology", *Science* 129: 303–7.

Campbell, J. B. 1994. *The Roman Army 31 BC–AD 337: A Sourcebook*. London: Routledge.

Caple, C. 2006. *Objects Reluctant Witnesses to the Past*. London: Routledge.

Carr, G. 2001. "Romanisation and the Body". In *Theoretical Roman Archaeology Conference Proceedings London 2000*, G. Davies, A. Gardner, and K. Lockyear, eds. Oxford: Oxbow Books, pp. 112–24.

Cech, B., ed. 2008. *Die Produktion von Ferrum Noricum am Hüttenberger Erzberg: die Ergebnisse der interdisziplinären Forschungen auf der Fundstelle Semlach. Eisner in den Jahren 2003–2005*. Wien: Österreichische Gesellschaft für Archäologie.

Charitonidou, A. 1978. *Epidauros: The Sanctuary of Asclepios*. Athens: Clio Editions.

Christie, N. 2011. *The Fall of the Western Roman Empire: An Archaeological and Historical Approach*. London: Bloomsbury Academic.

Ciaraldi, M. 1997. "Plant Remains". In *Anglo-American Pompeii Project 1996*, S. Bon, R. Jones, R. Kurchin, and D. Robinson, eds. Bradford: Archaeological Science Research 3, pp. 17–23.

2000. "Drug Preparation in Evidence? An Unusual Plant and Bone Assemblage from the Pompeian Countryside", *Vegetation History and Archaeobotany* 9: 91–8.

2002. "The Interpretation of Medicinal Plants in the Archaeological Context: Some Case Studies from Pompeii". *The Archaeology of Medicine Papers Given at the Session of the Annual Conference of the Theoretical Archaeology Group Held at the University of Birmingham on 20 December 1998*, R. Arnott, ed. Oxford: British Archaeological Reports International Series 1046, pp. 81–6.

Clark, J. G. D. 1939. *Archaeology and Society*. London: Methuen.

Clarke, D. 1973. "Archaeology: The Loss of Innocence", *Antiquity* 47: 6–18.

Clarke, J. R. 1998. *Looking at Lovemaking: Constructions of Sexuality in Roman Art: 100 BC to AD 250*. Berkeley: University of California Press.

Cockburn, A., E. Cockburn, and T. A. Reyman, eds. 1998 (2nd ed.). *Mummies, Diseases, and Ancient Cultures*. Cambridge: Cambridge University Press.

Conrad, L. 1995. "The Arab-Islamic Medical Tradition". In *The Western Medical Tradition 880 BC to AD 1800*, L. I. Conrad, M. Neve, V. Nutton, R. Porter, and A. Wear, eds. Cambridge: Cambridge University Press, pp. 93–138.

Conrad, L., M. Neve, V. Nutton, R. Porter, and A. Wear, eds. 1995. *The Western Medical Tradition 880 BC to AD 1800*. Cambridge: Cambridge University Press.

Cox, M. 2005. "Assessment of Age at Death and Sex in the Adult Human Skeleton". In *Handbook of Archaeological Sciences*, D. R. Brothwell and A. M. Pollard, eds. Chichester: John Wiley, pp. 237–48.

Crow, J. 1995. *Housesteads*. Bath: B. T. Batsford/English Heritage.

Crummy, P. 2002. "A Preliminary Account of the Doctor's Grave at Stanway, Colchester, England". In *Practitioners, Practices and Patients New Approaches to Medical Archaeology and*

Anthropology: Conference Proceedings, P. Baker and G. Carr, eds. Oxford: Oxbow Books, pp. 47–57.

Cruse, A. 2008 (2nd ed.). *Roman Medicine*. Stroud: Tempus.

Cüppers, H., ed. 1990. *Die Römer in Rheinland-Pfalz*. Stuttgart: Theiss.

Cuvigny, H. 2009. "The Finds of Papyri: The Archaeology of Papyri". In *The Oxford Handbook of Papyrology*, R. Bagnall, ed. Oxford: Oxford University Press, pp. 30–58.

Dasen, V. 1988. "Dwarfism in Egypt and Classical Antiquity: Iconography and Medical History", *Medical History* 32: 253–76.

   1993. *Dwarfs in Ancient Egypt and Greece*. Oxford: Clarendon Press.

   2008. "All Children Are Dwarfs: Medical Discourse and Iconography of Children's Bodies", *Oxford Journal of Archaeology* 27(1): 49–62.

Davies, R. 1969a. "Joining the Roman Army", *Bonner Jahrbücher* 169: 208–32.

   1969b. "The *Medici* of the Roman Armed Forces", *Epigraphische Studien* 8: 83–99.

Deetz, J. 1967. *Invitation to Archaeology*. Garden City, NY: Natural History Press.

   1977. *In Small Things Forgotten*. New York: Anchor Press/Doubleday.

   1996 (rev. ed.). *In Small Things Forgotten*. New York: Anchor Press/Doubleday.

Detys, S. 1988. "Les ex-voto de guerisons Gaule", *Dossiers Histoire et Archeolgie* 123: 82–7.

Diels, H. 1914. *Antike Technik*. Leipzig: B. G. Teubner.

Dyczek, P. 1995. "The *Valetudinarium* at Novae: New Components", *Acts of the 12th International Congress on Ancient Bronzes (NAR)*: 365–72.

Dyson, S. 1995. "Is There a Text in Site?" In *Historical and Archaeological Views on Texts and Archaeology*, D. Small, ed. Leiden: Brill, pp. 25–44.

Edelstein, E. J., and L. Edelstein 1988 [1945]. *Asclepius: Collection and Interpretation of the Testimonies*. Baltimore, MD: Johns Hopkins University Press.

Elderkin, G. W. 1911. "Tholos and Abaton at Epidauros", *American Journal of Archaeology* 15(2): 161–7.

Elsner, J. 1995. *Art and the Roman Viewer: The Transformation of Art from the Pagan World to Christianity*. Cambridge: Cambridge University Press.

Elsner, J., ed. 1996. *Art and Text in Roman Culture*. Cambridge: Cambridge University Press.

Evans, J., and T. O'Connor 1999. *Environmental Archaeology: Principles and Methods*. Stroud: Sutton.

Evershed, R. P., S. N. Dudd, M. J. Lockheart, and S. Jim 2005. "Lipids in Archaeology". In *Handbook of Archaeological Sciences*, D. R. Brothwell and A. M. Pollard, eds. Chichester: John Wiley, pp. 331–50.

Fagan, B. M. 1988 (3rd ed.). *Archaeology a Brief Introduction*. London: Scott, Foreman and Co.

Fagan, G. 1999. *Bathing in Public in the Roman World*. Ann Arbor: University of Michigan Press.

Faraone, C. A. 2009. "Stopping Evil, Pain, Anger, and Blood: The Ancient Greek Tradition of Protective Iambic Incantations". *Greek, Roman, and Byzantine Studies* 49: 227–55.

Filer, J. M. 1997. "Revealing Hermione's Secrets", *Egyptian Archaeology* 11: 32–4.

   1998. "Revealing the Face of Artemiodorus", *Minerva* 9(4): 21–4.

   1999. "Ein Blick der Menschen hinter den Portraits: eine Untersuchung agyptischer und Gesichtsrekonstruktion". In *Mummienportraits und agyptischer Grabkunst aus romischer Zeit*, K. Parlasca and H. Seemann, eds. Frankfurt: Schirn Kunsthalle, pp. 79–86.

   2002. "Ancient Bodies, but Modern Techniques. The Utilisation of CT Scanning in the Study of Ancient Egyptian Mummies". In *The Archaeology of Medicine Papers Given at the Session of the Annual Conference of the Theoretical Archaeology Group Held at the University of Birmingham on 20 December 1998*, R. Arnott, ed. Oxford: British Archaeological Reports International Series 1046, pp. 33–40.

Flemming, R. 2000. *Medicine and the Making of Roman Women*. Oxford: Oxford University Press.

Floriano, A. C. 1940–1941. "Aportaciones Arqueologicas a la Historia de la Medicina Romana", *Archivo Español de Arqueologia* 14: 415–33.

Frankfurter, D. 1994. "The Magic of Writing and the Writing of Magic: The Power of the Word in Egyptian and Greek Traditions", *Helios* 21: 189–221.

Frösén, J. 2009. "Conservation of Ancient Papyrus Materials". In *The Oxford Handbook of Papyrology*, R. Bagnall, ed. Oxford: Oxford University Press, pp. 79–100.

Gaffney, C., and J. Gater 2003. *Revealing the Buried Past: Geophysics for Archaeologists*. Stroud: Tempus.

Gaffney, V., Z. Stancic, and H. Watson 1995. "The Impact of GIS on Archaeology. A Personal Perspective". In *Archaeology and Geographical Information Systems*, G. Lock and Z. Stancic, eds. London: Taylor & Francis, pp. 319–34.

Gager, J. G. 1992. "Introduction". In *Curse Tablets and Binding Spells from the Ancient World*, J. G. Gager, ed. New York: Oxford University Press, pp. 3–33.

Galloway, P. 2006. "Material Culture and Text: Exploring the Spaces within and between". In *Historical Archaeology*, M. Hall and S. W. Silliman, eds. Oxford: Blackwell, pp. 42–64.

Gamble, C. 2004. *Archaeology the Basics*. London: Routledge.

  2008 (2nd ed.). *Archaeology the Basics*. London: Routledge.

Garland, R. 1995. *The Eye of the Beholder: Deformity and Disability in the Graeco-Roman World*. Ithaca, NY: Cornell University Press.

Gearney, A., E. R. Waite, M. J. Collins, O. E. Craig, and R. J. Sokol 2005. "Survival and Interpretation of Archaeological Proteins". In *Handbook of Archaeological Sciences*, D. R. Brothwell and A. M. Pollard, eds. Chichester: John Wiley, pp. 323–30.

Gell, A. 1994. "The Technology of Enchantment and the Enchantment of Technology". In *Anthropology, Art and Aesthetics*, J. Coote and A. Shelton, eds. Oxford: Clarendon Press, pp. 40–66.

Gero, J., and Conkey, M. W., eds. 2002. *Engendering Archaeology: Women and Prehistory*. Oxford: Basil Blackwell.

Gilchrist, R. 1994. *Gender and Material Culture: The Archaeology of Religious Women*. London: Routledge.

  1999. *Gender and Archaeology: Contesting the Past*. London: Routledge.

Gillings, M. 2005. "Spatial Information and Archaeology". In *Handbook of Archaeological Sciences*, D. R. Brothwell and A. M. Pollard, eds. Chichester: John Wiley, pp. 671–84.

Goldberg, M. Y. 1999. "Spatial and Behavioural Negotiation in Classical Athenian City Houses". In *The Archaeology of Household Activities*, P. M. Allison, ed. London: Routledge, pp. 142–61.

Gordon, A. E. 1983. *Illustrated Introduction to Latin Epigraphy*. Berkeley: University of California Press.

Gosden, G., and Y. Marshall 1999. "The Cultural Biography of Objects", *World Archaeology* 31(2): 169–78.

Green, C. M. C. 2004. *Roman Religion and the Cult of Diana at Aricia*. Cambridge: Cambridge University Press.

Green, M. 1992. *Dictionary of Celtic Myth and Legend*. London: Thames and Hudson.

Greene, K., and T. Moore 2010 (5th ed.). *Archaeology: An Introduction*. London: Routledge.

Grmek, M. 1988. "Les Affections de La Colonne Vertebrale dans L'iconographie medicale et les arts antiques", *Dossiers Histoire et Archéologie* 123: 52–61.

Grøn, O. 1991. "Introduction". In *Social Space: Human Spatial Behaviour in Dwellings and Settlements*, O. Grøn, E. Engelstad, and I. Lindblom, eds. Odense: Odense University Press, pp. 7–9.

Grøn, O., E. Engelstad, and I. Lindblom, eds. 1991. *Social Space: Human Spatial Behaviour in Dwellings and Settlements*. Odense: Odense University Press.

Gummerus, H. 1932. *Der Ärztesstand im römischen Reiche nach dem Inschriften*. Helsinki: Akademische Buchhandlung.

Harig, G. 1971. "Zum Problem „Krankenhaus" in der Antike", *Klio* 53: 179–95.

Harvey, K. 2009. "Introduction: Practical Matters". In *History and Material Culture: A Student's Guide to Approaching Alternative Sources*, K. Harvey, ed. London: Routledge, pp. 1–23.

Haynes, I. 1999. "Military Service and Cultural Identity in the *Auxilia*". In *The Roman Army as a Community*, A. Goldsworthy and I. Haynes, eds. Portsmouth, RI: Journal of Roman Archaeology Supplementary Series no. 34, pp. 165–74.

Heidegger, M. 1978. "Building Dwelling Thinking". In *Basic Writings*, D. F. Krell, ed. and trans. London: Routledge, pp. 319–39.

1993. "Building, Dwelling, Thinking". In *Basic Writings*, D. F. Krell, ed. and trans. San Francisco: Harper San Francisco, pp. 145–61.

Henderson, J. 2000. *The Science and Archaeology of Materials: An Investigation of Inorganic Materials*. London: Routledge.

Henig, M. 1995. *Handbook to Roman Art*. London: Phaidon Press.

2000. "From Classical Greece to Roman Britain: Some Hellenic Themes in Provincial Art and Glyptics". In *Periplous: Papers on Classical Art and Archaeology: To Sir John Boardman and his Pupils and Friends*, G. R. Tsetskhladze, A. M. Snodgrass, and A. J. N. W. Prag, eds. London: Thames and Hudson, pp. 124–35.

Hicks, D., and M. Beaudry, eds. 2006. *The Cambridge Companion to Historical Archaeology*. Cambridge: Cambridge University Press.

Hill, J. D. 1995. *Ritual and Rubbish in the Iron Age of Wessex*. Oxford: British Archaeological Reports, British Series 242.

Hingley, R. 1996. "The 'Legacy' of Rome: The Rise, Decline and Fall of the Theory of Romanisation". In *Roman Imperialism: Post-Colonial Perspectives*, J. Webster and N. Cooper, eds. Leicester: Leicester Archaeological Monographs No. 3, pp. 35–48.

2000. *Roman Officers and English Gentlemen: The Imperial Origins of Roman Archaeology*. London: Routledge.

Hodder, I. 1982a. *The Present Past: An Introduction to Anthropology for Archaeologists*. London: B. T. Batsford.

1982b. *Symbols in Action*. Cambridge: Cambridge University Press.

1996. *Theory and Practice in Archaeology*. London: Routledge.

2001. "Post-modernism, Post-structuralism and Post-processual Archaeology". In *The Meaning of Things: Material Culture and Symbolic Expression*, I. Hodder, ed. London: Harper Collins Academic, pp. 64–78.

2007 (7th ed.). *The Archaeological Process: An Introduction*. London: Blackwell.

Hodder, I., and S. Hutson 2003 (3rd ed.). *Reading the Past: Current Approaches to Interpretation in Archaeology*. Cambridge: Cambridge University Press.

Hodder, I., and R. Pruecel, eds. 1996. *Contemporary Archaeology in Theory*. Oxford: Blackwell.

Hodge, A. T. 1992. *Roman Aqueducts and Water Supply*. London: Duckworth.

Holden, T. G. 2005. "Dietary Evidence from the Coprolites and the Intestinal Contents of Ancient Humans". In *Handbook of Archaeological Sciences*, D. R. Brothwell and A. M. Pollard, eds. Chichester: John Wiley, pp. 403–25.

Hölscher, T. 2004. *The Language of Images in Roman Art*. Cambridge: Cambridge University Press.

Horden, P. 2008. *Hospitals and Healing from Antiquity to the Later Middle Ages*. Aldershot: Ashgate Variorum.

Houby-Nielsen, S. 2000. "Child Burials in Ancient Athens". In *Children and Material Culture*, J. Sofaer Derevenski, ed. London: Routledge, pp. 151–66.

Hughes, J. 2008. "Fragmentation as Metaphor in the Classical Healing Sanctuary", *Social History of Medicine* 21(2): 217–36.

Huisman, F., and J. H. Warner 2004. "Medical Histories". In *Locating Medical History: The Stories and their Meanings*, F. Huisman and J. H. Warner, eds. Baltimore, MD: Johns Hopkins University Press, pp. 1–30.

Hunt, P. 2005. *Aeneid XII. 383–440 as Inspiration for Ancient Art: The Roman Surgeon*. http://traumwerk.stanford.edu/philolog/2005/11/aeneid_as_inspiration_for_anci.html

Hurcombe, L. 2007. *Archaeological Artefacts as Material Culture*. London: Routledge.

Ingold, T. 1993. "The Temporality of Landscape", *World Archaeology* 25(2): 152–73.

Jackson, R. 1988. *Doctors and Diseases in the Roman Empire*. London: British Museum Publications.

1990a. "Roman Doctors and their Instruments: Recent Research into Ancient Practice", *Journal of Roman Archaeology* 3: 5–27.

1990b. "Waters and Spas in the Classical World". In *The Medical History of Waters and Spas*, R. Porter, ed. London: Wellcome Institute for the History of Medicine, pp. 1–13.

1993. "Roman Medicine: Practitioners and their Practices". In *Aufstieg und Niedergang der Romischen Welt* II 37.1, H. Temporini and W. Haase, ed. Berlin: Walter de Gruyter, pp. 79–100.

1994a. "The Mouse, the Lion and the Crooked One: Two Enigmatic Roman Handle Types", *The Antiquaries Journal* 74: 325–32.

1994b. "Styphylagra, Staphylocaustes, Uvulectomy and Haemorrhoidectomy: The Roman Instruments and Operations". In *From Epidauros toSalerno: Symposium Held at the European University Centre for Cultural Heritage, Ravello, April 1990*, A. Krug, ed. Rixensart: Pact Belgium, pp. 167–85.

1994c. "The Surgical Instruments, Appliances and Equipment in Celsus' *De Medicina*". In *La Médecine de Celse*, G. Sabbah and J. Mundry, eds. Saint-Étienne: Publications de l'Université Saint-Étienne, pp. 167–209.

1995. "The Composition of Roman Medical *Instrumentaria* as an Indicator of Medical Practice: A Provisional Assessment". In *Ancient Medicine in its Socio-cultural Context*, Ph. J. van der Eijk, H. F. J. Horstmanshoff, and P. H. Schrijvers, eds. Amsterdam: Rodopi Press, pp. 189–208.

1996. "Eye Medicine in the Roman Empire". In *Aufstieg und Niedergang der Romischen Welt* II 37.3, H. Temporini and W. Haase, eds. Berlin: Walter de Gruyter, pp. 2228–51.

1997. "An Ancient British Medical Kit from Stanway, Essex". *The Lancet* 350(9089): 1471–3.

2002. "Roman Surgery: The Evidence of the Instruments". In *The Archaeology of Medicine Papers Given at the Session of the Annual Conference of the Theoretical Archaeology Group Held at the University of Birmingham on 20 December 1998*, R. Arnott, ed. Oxford: British Archaeological Reports International Series 1046, pp. 87–94.

2005. "Holding on to Health? Bone Surgery and Instrumentation in the Roman Empire". In *Health in Antiquity*, H. King, ed. London: Routledge, pp. 97–119.

2007. "The Surgical Instruments". In *Stanway: An Élite Burial Site at Camulodunum*, P. Crummy, S. Benfield, N. Crummy, V. Rigby, and D. Shimmin, eds. Britannia Monograph Series no. 24. London: Society for the Promotion of Roman Studies, pp. 236–52.

James, S. 1999. "The Community of Soldiers: A Major Identity and Centre of Power in the Roman Empire". In *TRAC 98: Proceedings of the Eighth Annual Theoretical Roman Archaeology Conference, Leicester 1998*, P. Baker, C. Forcey, S. Jundi, and R. Witcher, eds. Oxford: Oxbow Books, pp. 14–25.

2002. "Writing the Legions: The Development and Future of Roman Military Studies in Britain", *Archaeological Journal* 159: 1–58.

Jameson, M. H. 1990. "Domestic Space in the Greek City State". In *Domestic Architecture and the Use of Space: An Interdisciplinary and Cross-Cultural Study*, S. Kent, eds. Cambridge: Cambridge University Press, pp. 92–113.

Jansen, G. C. M. 1997. "Private Toilets at Pompeii: Appearance and Operation". In *Sequence and Space in Pompeii*, S. E. Bon and R. Jones, eds. Oxford: Oxbow Books, pp. 121–34.

Jettner, D. 1966. *Geschichte des Hospitals*. Sudhoffs Archive für Geschichte der Medizin und der Naturwissenschaften 11. Wiesbaden: Franz Steiner Verlag GmbH.

Johnson, A. 1983. *Roman Forts*. London: Adam and Charles Black.

Johnson, M. 2000. *Archaeological Theory: An Introduction*. Oxford: Blackwell.

2007. *Ideas of Landscape*. Oxford: Blackwell.

2009 (2nd ed.). *Archaeological Theory: An Introduction*. Oxford: Blackwell.

Jones, Andrew. 2002. *Archaeological Theory and Scientific Practice*. Cambridge: Cambridge University Press.

Jones, Alexander. 2009. "Mathematics, Science and Medicine in Papyri". In *The Oxford Handbook of Papyrology*, R. Bagnall, ed. Oxford: Oxford University Press, pp. 338–57.

Kent, S. 1990. "Activity Areas and Architecture: An Interdisciplinary View of the Relationship between Use of Space and Domestic Built Environment". In *Domestic Architecture and the Use of Space: An Interdisciplinary Cross-Cultural Study*, S. Kent, ed. Cambridge: Cambridge University Press, pp. 1–8.

Keppie, L. 1991. *Understanding Roman Inscriptions*. London: B. T. Batsford.

King, H. 2001. *Greek and Roman Medicine*. Bristol: Bristol Classical Press.

Kleiner, D. E. E. 1992. *Roman Sculpture*. New Haven, CT: Yale University Press.

Kleinman, A. 1980. *Patients and Healers in the Context of Culture*. Berkeley: University of California Press.

Koenen, C. 1904. "Beschreibung von Novaesium", *Bonner Jahrbucher* 111/112: 97–242.

Koloski-Ostrow, A. O. 1996. "Finding Social Meaning in the Public Latrines of Pompeii". In *Cura Aquarum in Campania*, N. de Haan and G. C. M Jansen, eds. Leiden: Brill, pp. 79–86.

Kraay, M. H. 1966. *Greek Coins*. London: Thames and Hudson.

Künzl, E. 1979/81. "Medizinische Instrumente aus dem römischen Altertum in Städtischen Museum Worms", *Der Wormsgau* 13: 49–63.

   1982. "Römische Medizin im Spiegel archäologischer Funde", *Archäologie in Deutschland* 1(Jan–März) 14.

   1983a. *Medizinische Instrumente aus Sepulkralfunden der römischen Kaiserzeit*. Cologne: Rheinland Verlag GmbH.

   1983b. "Was soll die Maus auf dem chirurgischen Instrument?" In *Antidoron Festschrift Jürgen Thimme zum 65 Geburtstag am 26. September 1982*, J. Thimme, D. Metzler, B. Otto, and C. Müller-Wirth, eds. Karlsruhe: C. F. Müller, pp. 111–16.

   1984. "Einige Bemerkungen zu den Herstellern der romischen medizinischen Instrumente", *Alba Regia* 21: 59–65.

   1984/5. "Der Schropfkopf vom Limeskastell Zugmantel", *Saalburg Jahrbuch* 40/41: 30–3.

   1986. "Operationsräume in römischen Thermen", *Bonner Jahrbücher* 186: 491–509.

   1989/90. "Römisches Thermen als Spitäler", *Römisches Österreich* 17/18: 147–52.

   1996. "Forschungsbericht zu den antiken medizinischen Instrumenten". In *Aufstieg und Niedergang der Romischen Welt* II 37.3, H. Temporini and W. Haase, eds. Berlin: Walter de Gruyter, pp. 2433–639.

   2002. *Medizin in der Antike: aus einer Welt ohne Narkose und Aspirin*. Stuttgart: Konrad Theiss Verlag GmbH.

Lang, M. 1977. *Cure and Cult in Ancient Corinth. American Excavations in Old Corinth Series Corinth Notes, No. 1*. Princeton, NJ: American School of Classical Studies at Athens.

Laqueur, T. W. 1990. *Making Sex: Body and Gender from the Greeks to Freud*. Cambridge, MA: Harvard University Press.

Larsen, C. S. 1997. *Bioarchaeology: Interpreting Behaviour from the Human Skeleton*. Cambridge: Cambridge University Press.

Laurence, R. 2007 (2nd ed.). *Roman Pompeii: Space and Society*. London: Routledge.

   2012. *Roman Archaeology for Historians*. London: Routledge.

Leven, K.-H. 2004. "At times these ancient facts seem to lie before me like a patient on a hospital bed" – Retrospective Diagnosis and Ancient Medical History. In *Magi and Rationality in Ancient Near Eastern and Graeco-Roman Medicine*, H. F. J. Horstmanshoff, M. Stol, and C. van Tilburg, eds. Leiden: Brill, pp. 369–86.

Ling, R. 1991. *Roman Painting*. Cambridge: Cambridge University Press.

Little, L. 1999. "Abstract: Babies in Well G5:3: Preliminary Results and Future Analysis", *American Journal of Archaeology* 103(1): 284.

Majno, G. 1975. *The Healing Hand*. Cambridge, MA: Harvard University Press.

Mattingly, D. 1997. "Introduction: Dialogues of Power and Experience in the Roman Empire". In *Dialogues, Discourse and Discrepant Experiences in the Roman Empire*, D. Mattingly, ed. Portsmouth, RI: Journal of Roman Archaeology Supplementary Series no. 23, pp. 7–24.

Mauss, M. 1979 [1936]. "Techniques of the Body", *Economy and Society* 2: 70–88.

Mays, S. 1998. *The Archaeology of Human Bones*. London: Routledge.

McDonald, G. 2012. "The 'Locus Affectus' in Ancient Medical Theories of Disease". In *Body, Buildings and Space in the Classical and Medieval Islamic and Western Traditions*, Proceedings of the Anglo-Dutch Wellcome Symposium, Nijmegen, November 2007, P. Baker, H. Nijdam, and C. van't Land, eds. Leiden: Brill, pp. 63–84.

McKinley, J. I., and J. M. Bond 2005. "Cremated Bone". In *Handbook of Archaeological Sciences*, D. R. Brothwell and A. M. Pollard, eds. Chichester: John Wiley, pp. 281–92.

Melas, A. M. 2001. "Etics, Emics and the Empathy in Archaeological Theory". In *The Meaning of Things: Material Culture and Symbolic Expression*, I. Hodder, ed. London: Routledge, pp. 137–55.

Merleau-Ponty, M. 1962. *Phenomenology of Perception*, Colin Smith, trans. London: Routledge & Kegan Paul.

Meskell, L. M. 1994. "Dying Young: The Experience of Death at Deir el Medina", *Archaeological Review from Cambridge* 13: 35–45.

Metzler, I. 2012. "Liminality and Disability: Spatial and Conceptual Aspects of Physical Impairment in Medieval Europe". In *Medicine and Space: Body, Surroundings and Borders in Antiquity and the Middle Ages*, Proceedings of the Anglo-Dutch Wellcome Symposium, Nijmegen, November 2007, P. Baker, H. Nijdam, and C. van't Land, eds. Leiden: Brill, pp. 273–96.

Millett, M. 1990a. "Romanization: Historical Issues and Archaeological Interpretation". In *The Early Roman Empire in the West*, T. Blagg and M. Millett, eds. Oxford: Oxbow Books, pp. 35–41.

1990b. *The Romanization of Britain: An Essay in Archaeological Interpretation*. Cambridge: Cambridge University Press.

2007. "Roman Archaeology". In *Classical Archaeology*, S. E. Alcock and R. Osborne, eds. Oxford: Blackwell, pp. 30–50.

Milne, J. 1907. *Surgical Instruments in Greek and Roman Times*. Oxford: Clarendon Press.

Molina, M. 1981. "Instrumental Medico de Epoca Romana en el Museo Arqueologico Nacional (Madrid)", *Archivo Español de Arqueologia* 55: 255–62.

Molleson, T., and M. Cox 1988. "A Neonate with Cut Bones from Poundbury Camp, 4th Century AD, England", *Bulletin de la Société royal Belge d'Anthropologie et de Préhistoire* 99: 53–9.

Moore, H. L. 1982. "The Interpretation of Spatial Patterning in Settlement Residues". In *Symbolic and Structural Archaeology*, I. Hodder, ed. Cambridge: Cambridge University Press, pp. 74–9.

1996. *Space, Text and Gender: An Anthropological Study of the Marakwet of Kenya*. New York: Guilford Press.

Moreland, J. 2007. *Archaeology and Text*. London: Duckworth.

Morphy, H., and M. Perkins 2006. "The Anthropology of Art: A Reflection on its History and Contemporary Practice". In *The Anthropology of Art: A Reader*, H. Morphy and M. Perkins, eds. Oxford: Blackwell, pp. 1–32.

Neudecker, R. 1994. *Die Pracht der Latrine: Zum Wandel öffentlicher Bedürfnisanstalten in der kaiserzeitlichen Stadt*. Munich: F. Pfeil.

Nicholls, M. 2010. "Parchment Codices in the New Text of Galen", *Greece and Rome* 57(2): 378–86.

2011. "Galen and Libraries in the *Peri Alupias*", *Journal of Roman Studies* 101: 123–42.

Nutton, V. 1969. "Medicine and the Roman Army: A Further Reconsideration", *Medical History* 13: 260–70.

1972. "Roman Oculists", *Epigraphica* 34: 16–29.

2004. *Ancient Medicine*. London: Routledge.

2009. "Galen's Library". In *Galen and the World of Knowledge*, C. Gill, T. Whitmarsh, and J. Wilkins, eds. Cambridge: Cambridge University Press, pp. 19–34.

Ober, J. 1995. "Greek Horoi: Artifactual Texts and the Contingency of Meaning". In *Historical and Archaeological Views on Texts and Archaeology*, D. Small, ed. Leiden: Brill, pp. 91–123.

O'Connor, T. P. 2004. *The Archaeology of Animal Bones*. Stroud: Sutton.

Oosten, J. 1992. "Representing the Spirits: The Mask of the Alaskan Inuit". In *Anthropology Art and Aesthetics*, J. Coote and A. Shelton, eds. Oxford: Clarendon Press, pp. 113–36.

Ortner, D. J. 2005. "Disease Ecology". In *Handbook of Archaeological Sciences*, D. R. Brothwell and A. M. Pollard, eds. Chichester: John Wiley, pp. 225–36.

Ortner, S. B., and H. Whitehead 1981. *Sexual Meanings and the Cultural Construction of Gender and Sexuality*. Cambridge: Cambridge University Press.

Panayotatou, A. G. 1919. "Baths and Bathing in Ancient Greece", *Proceedings of the Royal Society of Medicine* 12(suppl.): 107–21.

Papadopoulos, J. K. 2000, "Skeletons in Wells: Towards an Archaeology of Social Exclusions in the Ancient Greek World". In *Madness, Disability and Social Exclusion: The Archaeology and Anthropology of Difference*, J. Hubert, ed. London: Routledge, pp. 98–118.

Parker Pearson, M., and C. Richards 1994. "Ordering the World: Perceptions of Architecture, Space and Time". In *Architecture and Order: Approaches to Social Space*, M. Parker Pearson and C. Richards, eds. London: Routledge, pp. 1–37.

Pedley, J. G. 1998 (2nd ed.). *Greek Art and Archaeology*. London: Laurence King.

Penn, R. G. 1994. *Medicine on Ancient Greek and Roman Coins*. London: B. T. Batsford.

Perring, D., and Brigham, T. 2000. "Londinium and its Hinterland: The Roman Period". In *The Archaeology of Greater London. An Assessment of Archaeological Evidence for Human Presence in the Area Now Covered by Greater London*, M. Kendall, ed. Suffolk: MoLAS Monograph, Museum of London, pp. 120–70.

Pollard, J. 2001. "The Aesthetics of Depositional Practice", *World Archaeology* 33(2): 315–33.

Pollitt, J. J. 1972. *Art and Experience in Classical Greece*. Cambridge: Cambridge University Press.

Praetzellis, A. 2003. *Dug to Death: A Tale of Archaeological Method and Mayhem*. New York: Altamira Press.

   2011 (rev. ed.). *Death by Theory: A Tale of Mystery and Archaeological Theory*. New York: Altamira Press.

Preucel, R. W., and L. Meskell 2007. "Places". In *A Companion to Social Archaeology*, L. Meskell and R. W. Preucel, eds. Oxford: Blackwell, pp. 215–29.

Raddatz, K. 1973. *Mulva I. Die Grabungen in der Nekropole in den Jahren 1957 und 1958*. Mainz: Verlag Philipp von Zabern (Madrider Beiträge).

Ramage, N. H., and A. Ramage 2000. *Roman Art*. London: Laurence King.

Rankov, B. 2004. "Breaking Down Boundaries: The Experience of the Multidisciplinary Olympias Project". In *Archaeology and Ancient History: Breaking Down the Boundaries*, E. W. Sauer, ed. London: Routledge, pp. 49–61.

Rapoport, A. 1969. *House, Form and Culture*. Englewood Cliffs, NJ: Prentice Hall.

   1990. "Systems of Activities and Systems of Settings". In *Domestic Architecture and the Use of Space and Interdisciplinary Cross-Cultural Study*, S. Kent, ed. Cambridge: Cambridge University Press, pp. 9–20.

Redfern, R. 2003. "Sex and the City: A Biocultural Investigation into Female Health in Roman Britain". In *TRAC 2002: Proceedings of the Twelfth Annual Theoretical Roman Archaeology Conference, Canterbury 2002*, G. Carr, E. Swift, and J. Weekes, eds. Oxford: Oxbow Books, pp. 147–70.

Redknap, M., G. Clarke, M. Henig, M. R. Hull, D. Peacock, J. Shepherd, V. Snetterton-Lewis, and Jane Timby 1986. "The Small Finds". In *Excavations on the Romano-British Small Town at Neatham, Hampshire*, M. Millett and D. Graham, eds. Farnham: Hampshire Field Club and Farnham and District Museum Societies, pp. 101–39.

Reithmüller, J. W. 2005. *Asklepios: Heiligtümer und Kulte*. Heidelberg: Verlag Archäologie und Geschichte.

Rémy, B. 1984. "Les Inscriptions de médecins en Gaule", *Gallia* 42: 115–52.

   1991. "Les Inscriptions de médicines dans les provinces romaines de la péninsule ibérique", *REA* 93: 321–64.

Rémy, B., and P. Faure 2010. *Les Médecines dans l'Occident romain: Péninsule Ibérique, Bregtagne, Gaules, Germaines*. Paris: Ausonius Publications: Scripta Antiqua 27, Ausonius, Pessac/Diffusion de Boccard.

Renfrew, C., and P. Bahn 2005. *Archaeology: The Key Concepts*. London: Routledge.

   2008 (5th ed.). *Archaeology: Theories, Methods and Practices*. London: Thames and Hudson.

Revel, L. 2005. "The Roman Life Course: A View from the Inscriptions", *European Journal of Archaeology* 8(1): 43–63.

Reynolds, L. D., and N. G. Wilson 1978 (2nd ed.). *Scribes and Scholars: A Guide to the Transmission of Greek and Latin Literature*. Oxford: Oxford University Press.

Richards, C., and J. Thomas 1984. "Ritual Activity and Structured Deposition in Later Neolithic Wessex". In *Neolithic Studies: A Review of Some Current Research*, R. Bradley and J. Gardiner, eds. Oxford: British Archaeological Reports, British Series 133, pp. 198–218.

Roberts, C. A. 1988. "Trauma and Treatment in British Antiquity: A Radiographic Study". In *Science and Archaeology. Glasgow 1987*, E. Slater and J. Tate, eds. Oxford: British Archaeological Reports British Series 96(ii), pp. 339–59.

2002. "Paleopathology and Archaeology: The Current State of Play". In *The Archaeology of Medicine Papers Given at the Session of the Annual Conference of the Theoretical Archaeology Group Held at the University of Birmingham on 20 December 1998*, R. Arnott, ed. Oxford: British Archaeological Reports International Series 1046, pp. 1–20.

2009. *Human Remains in Archaeology: A Handbook*. York: Council for British Archaeology.

Roberts, C. A., and J. Buikstra 2003. *The Bioarchaeology of Tuberculosis: A Global View on a Reemerging Disease*. Gainsville: University of Florida Press.

Roberts, C. A., and K. Manchester 2005. *The Archaeology of Disease*. Stroud: Sutton.

Roberts, C. A., and M. Cox 2003. *Health and Disease in Britain: From Prehistory to the Present Day*. Stroud: Sutton.

Roberts, C. A., and S. Ingham 2008. "Using Ancient DNA Analysis in Palaeopathology: A Critical Analysis of Published Papers with Recommendations for Future Work", *International Journal of Osteoarchaeology* 18: 600–13.

Robinson, M. 2005. "Insects as Palaeoenvironmental Indicators". In *Handbook of Archaeological Sciences*, D. R. Brothwell and A. M. Pollard, eds. Chichester: John Wiley, pp. 121–33.

Rosen, R. 2012. "Spaces of Sickness in Greco-Roman Medicine". In *Body, Buildings and Space in the Classical and Medieval Islamic and Western Traditions*, Proceedings of the Anglo-Dutch Wellcome Symposium, Nijmegen, November 2007, P. Baker, H. Nijdam, and C. van't Land, eds. Leiden: Brill, pp. 227–44.

Roskams. S. 2001. *Excavation*. Cambridge: Cambridge University Press.

Rowsome, P. 2000. *Heart of the City: Roman, Medieval and Modern London Revealed by Archaeology at 1 Poultry*. London: English Heritage, Museum of London Archaeological Service.

Rushworth, A. 2009. *Housesteads Roman Fort – The Grandest Station (Vols 1 and 2)*. Swindon: English Heritage.

Salazar, C. 2000. *The Treatment of War Wounds in Graeco-Roman Antiquity*. Leiden: Brill.

Salles, C. 1988. "Les Cachets D'Oculistes: Des ordonnances sur la Pierre", *Dossiers Histoire et Archaeologie* 126: 62–4.

Sauer, E. W., ed. 2004. *Archaeology and Ancient History: Breaking Down the Boundaries*. London: Routledge.

Scarborough, J. 1968. "Roman Medicine and the Legions: A Reconsideration", *Medical History* 12: 254–61.

1976. *Roman Medicine*. Ithaca, NY: Cornell University Press.

1977. "Some Beetles in Pliny's *Natural History*", *Coleopterist's Bulletin* 31: 293–96.

1978. "Theophrastus on Herbals and Herbal Remedies", *Journal of the History of Biology* 11, 353–85.

1983. "Theoretical Assumptions in Hippocratic Pharmacology". In *Formes de pensées dans la collection hippocratique: actes du IVe-Coloque-International) Hippocratique (Lausanne, 21–26 septembre 1981)*, F. Lasserre and P. Mudry, eds. Geneva: Librairie Droz, pp. 307–25.

2010. *Pharmacy and Drug Lore in Antiquity: Greece, Rome and Byzantium*. Farnham: Ashgate.

Scheuer, L., and S. Black 2000. *Developmental Juvenile Osteology*. Cambridge: Cambridge University Press.

Schnapp, A. 1996. *The Discovery of the Past: The Origins of Archaeology*. London: British Museum Press.

Scott, E. 1991. "Animal and Infant Burials in Romano-British Villas: A Revitalization Movement". In *Sacred and Profane Proceedings of a Conference on Archaeology, Ritual and Religion, Oxford 1989*, P. Garwood, D. Jennings, R. Skeates, and J. Toms, eds. Oxford: Oxford University Committee for Archaeology, pp. 116–19.

Scott, E., ed. 1993. *Theoretical Roman Archaeology: First Conference Proceedings*. Avebury: Aldershot.

Scott, S., and J. Webster, eds. 2003. *Roman Imperialism and Provincial Art*. Cambridge: Cambridge University Press.

Sealy, J. 2005. "Body Tissue Chemistry and the Paleodiet". In *Handbook of Archaeological Sciences*, D. R. Brothwell and A. M. Pollard, eds. Chichester: John Wiley, pp. 269–80.

Sear, D. R. 1978/9. *Greek Coins and their Values*, Vols. 1–2. London: Seaby.

    1988. *Roman Coins and Their Values*. London: Seaby.

Shanks, M. 1995. *Classical Archaeology of Greece: Experiences of the Discipline*. London: Routledge.

Shanks, M., and C. Tilley 1987. *Social Theory in Archaeology*. Cambridge: Polity Press.

    1992. *Reconstructing Archaeology, Theory and Practice*. London: Routledge.

Shennan, S. 1996. "Cultural Transmission and Cultural Change". In *Contemporary Archaeology in Theory*, R. W. Preucel and I. Hodder, eds. Oxford: Blackwell, pp. 282–96.

Small, D., ed. 1995a. *Historical and Archaeological Views on Texts and Archaeology*. Leiden: Brill.

Small, D. 1995b. "Monuments, Laws, and Analysis: Combining Archaeology and Text in Ancient Athens". In *Historical and Archaeological Views on Texts and Archaeology*, D. Small, ed. Leiden: Brill, pp. 143–74.

Smith, P. R., and M. T. Wilson 2005. "Blood Residues in Archaeology". In *Handbook of Archaeological Sciences*, D. R. Brothwell and A. M. Pollard, eds. Chichester: John Wiley, pp. 313–22.

Snodgrass, A. 2007. "Greek Archaeology". In *Classical Archaeology*, S. E. Alcock and R. Osborne, eds. Oxford: Blackwell, pp. 13–29.

Sofaer, J. 2006. *The Body as Material Culture: A Theoretical Osteoarchaeology*. Cambridge: Cambridge University Press.

Start, M. 2002. "Morbid Osteology". In *The Archaeology of Medicine Papers Given at the Session of the Annual Conference of the Theoretical Archaeology Group Held at the University of Birmingham on 20 December 1998*, R. Arnott, ed. Oxford: British Archaeological Reports International Series 1046, pp. 113–24.

Stewart, A. 1997. *Art, Desire and the Body in Ancient Greece*. Cambridge: Cambridge University Press.

Strathern, A. J. 1999. *Body Thoughts*. Ann Arbor: University of Michigan Press.

Susini, G. 1973. *The Roman Stonecutter: An Introduction to Latin Epigraphy*. A. M. Dabrowski, trans. Oxford: Basil Blackwell.

Tarlow, S. 1999. "Strangely Familiar". In *The Familiar Past: Archaeologies of Later Historical Britain*, S. Tarlow and S. West, eds. London: Routledge, pp. 263–72.

Taylor, G. M., P. Rutland, and T. Molleson 1997. "A Sensitive Polymerase Chain Reaction Method for the Protection of *Plasmodium* Species DNA in Ancient Remains", *Ancient Biomolecules* 1: 193–203.

Thomas, J. C. 1990. "Some other Analogy". In *Writing in the Past*, F. Baker and J. Thomas, eds. Lampeter: St. David's University Press, pp. 18–24.

    1991. *Rethinking the Neolithic*. Cambridge: Cambridge University Press.

Tilley, C. 1994. *A Phenomenology of Landscape: Places, Paths, and Monuments*. Oxford: Berg.

    1999. *Metaphor and Material Culture*. Oxford: Blackwell.

    2001. "Interpreting Material Culture". In *The Meaning of Things: Material Culture and Symbolic Expression*, I. Hodder, ed. London: Routledge, pp. 184–94.

    2002. "Metaphor, Materiality and Interpretation". In *The Material Culture Reader*, V. Bucchli, ed. Oxford: Berg, pp. 23–56.

Tobin, R. 1975. "The Canon of Polykleitos", *American Journal of Archaeology* 74(4): 307–21.

Tomlin, R. 2002. "Writing to the Gods in Britain". In *Becoming Roman, Writing Latin? Literacy and Epigraphy in the Roman West*, A. E. Cooley, ed. Portsmouth, RI: Journal of Roman Archaeology Supplementary Series no. 48, pp. 165–79.

Tomlinson, R. A. 1983. *Epidauros*. Austin: University of Texas Press.

Totelin, L. 2009. *Hippocratic Recipes: Oral and Written Transmission of Pharmacological Knowledge in Fifth- and Fourth-Century Greece*. Leiden: Brill.

Trigger, B. 2006 (2nd ed.). *A History of Archaeological Thought*. Cambridge: Cambridge University Press.

Tucci, P. L. 2008. "Galen's Storeroom, Rome's Libraries, and the Fire of A.D. 192", *Journal of Roman Archaeology* 21: 133–49.

Turner, B. S. 1984. *The Body and Society*. Oxford: Sage.

van der Veen, M. 2011. *Consumption, Trade and Intervention: Exploring the Botanical Remains from the Roman and Islamic Ports at Quseir al-Qadim, Egypt*. Frankfurt: Africa Magna Verlag.

van Driel-Murray, C., and M. Gechter 1984. *Funde aus der Fabrica der legio I Minerva am Bonner Berg. Beiträge zur Archäologie des Romischen Rheinlands 4*. Cologne: Rheinland-Verlag GmbH.

Vermeule, E. 1996. "Archaeology and Philology: The Dirt and the Word", *Transactions of the American Philological Association* 126: 1–10.

Versnel, H. S. 2002. "The Poetics of the Magical Charm: An Essay on the Power of Words". In *Magic and Ritual in the Ancient World*, O. P. Mirecki and M. Meyer, eds. Leiden: Brill, pp. 105–58.

Vickers, M., and D. Gill 1994. *Artful Crafts: Ancient Greek Silverware and Pottery*. Oxford: Clarendon Press.

Voinot, J. 1999. *Les Cachets à Collyres dans le Monde Romain*. Montagnac: Monique Mergoil (Instrumentum 7).

von Petrikovitz, H. 1975. *Die Innenbauten römischer Legionslager während der Prinzipatzeit*. Berlin: Westdeutscher Verlag.

Wallace-Hadrill, A. 2007. "The Roman World". In *Classical Archaeology*, S. E. Alcock and R. Osborne, eds. Oxford: Blackwell, pp. 355–80.

Watson, G. R. 1969. *The Roman Soldier*. Ithaca, NY: Cornell University Press.

Webster, J. 1996. "Sanctuaries and Sacred Places". In *The Celtic World*, M. Green, ed. London: Routledge, pp. 445–64.

    1997a. "Necessary Comparisons: A Post-Colonial Approach to Religious Syncretism in the Roman Provinces", *World Archaeology* 28(3): 324–38.

    1997b. "A Negotiated Syncretism: Readings on the Development of Romano-Celtic Religion". In *Dialogues in Roman Imperialism*, D. Mattingly, ed. Portsmouth, RI: Journal of Roman Archaeology Supplementary Series no. 23, pp. 165–84.

Weiss, E. 2009. *Bioarchaeological Science: What We Have Learned from Human Skeletal Remains*. New York: Nova Science.

Wells, C. 1985. "A Medical Interpretation of the Votive Terracottas: An Appendix to T. Potter's A Republican Healing-Sanctuary at Ponte di Nona near Rome and the Classical Tradition of Votive Medicine", *Journal of the British Archaeological Association* 138: 41–4.

Wells, P. S. 1999. *The Barbarians Speak: How the Conquered Peoples Shaped Roman Europe*. Princeton, NJ: Princeton University Press.

Whitley, J. 2001. *The Archaeology of Ancient Greece*. Cambridge: Cambridge University Press.

Wilkinson, K., and C. Stevens 2005. *Environmental Archaeology: Approaches, Techniques and Applications*. Stroud: Tempus.

Williams, D. 1983. "Women on Athenian Vases: Problems of Interpretation". In *Images of Women in Antiquity-1*, A. Cameron, ed. London: Croom Helm, pp. 92–106.

Wilmanns, J. C. 1995. *Der Sanitätsdienst im römischen Reich*. Medizin der Antike (2). Hildesheim: Olms Weidmann.

Winckelmann, J. J. 1764. *Geschicte der Kunst des Alterthums*. Dresden: Waltherische hof-Buchhandlung.

Woolf, G. 1998. *Becoming Roman: The Origins of Provincial Civilization in Gaul*. Cambridge: Cambridge University Press.

    2003. "Seeing Apollo in Roman Gaul and Germany". In *Roman Imperialism and Provincial Art*, S. Scott and J. Webster, eds. Cambridge: Cambridge University Press, pp. 139–52.

Yegül, F. 1992. *Baths and Bathing in Classical Antiquity*. Cambridge, MA: Harvard University Press.

Zacharia, K., ed. 2008. *Hellenisms: Culture, Identity, and Ethnicity from Antiquity to Modernity*. Aldershot: Ashgate.

Zanker, P. 1990. *The Power of Images in the Age of Augustus*, A. Shapiro, trans. Ann Arbor: University of Michigan Press.

Zienkiewicz, J. D. 1986. *The Legionary Fortress Baths at Caerleon II: The Finds*. Cardiff: Cadw, Welsh Historical Monuments.

Zimmerman, M. R. 2005. "The Study of Preserved Human Tissue". In *Handbook of Archaeological Sciences*, D. R. Brothwell and A. M. Pollard, eds. Chichester: John Wiley, pp. 249–57.

INDEX

For EU product safety concerns, contact us at Calle de José Abascal, 56–1°,
28003 Madrid, Spain or eugpsr@cambridge.org.